Marketing implant dentistry

To my wife Sandra, and children Morgan and Myles. Thank you for your patience and unwavering support of this project. To my father Walter Hines, Sr. and late mother Fay Hines, thank you for the positive examples and countless sacrifices you made so that I may spread my wings and fly. To my brother Dr. Daniel Hines who gave me my first job in dentistry.

Marketing implant dentistry

Attract and influence patients to accept your dental implant treatment plan

Marcus Hines

Director, Full Arch Solutions
BioHorizons Implant Systems, Inc.
Birmingham, AL, USA

WILEY Blackwell

Library of Congress Cataloging-in-Publication Data:

Hines, Marcus, author.
 Marketing implant dentistry : attract and influence patients to accept your dental implant treatment plan / Marcus Hines.
   p. ; cm.
 Includes bibliographical references and index.
 ISBN 978-1-119-11451-2 (cloth)
 I. Title.
 [DNLM: 1. Dental Implantation–economics. 2. Marketing of Health Services–methods. 3. Audiovisual Aids–standards. 4. Dental Implants–economics. 5. Internet–standards. WU 640]
 RK667.I45
 617.6'9300688–dc23

                                                                                           2015018035

Cover image: Front cover illustration: Leonard Morgan.
            Background illustration: designed by Freepik.com

Set in 10.5/13.5pt Meridien by SPi Global, Pondicherry, India

1   2016

Contents

Foreword

Talented clinicians have realized that there are a group of patients who should have been premier implant patients in their practices. This is often based on the car the patient drives, the community they live in, their children's private education, vacation homes, and the like.

Unfortunately, many of these patients refuse the implant options presented to them, or even seek implant treatment at treatment centers that may market well, but do not necessarily provide the highest level of care.

The question becomes, "Why do patients refuse implant treatment plans due to 'financial reasons' or seek treatment elsewhere?"

Implant treatment is a value-based service. Success comes from combining high levels of clinical expertise with the ability to communicate not only a complex process but also the value to the patient that comes along with receiving treatment at your practice.

Established clinicians should not ignore the importance of solid internal marketing. A typical practice's existing patient population can be one of the most reliable sources of generating new implant cases for any practice.

Most offices don't maximize their own abundant database of patients with missing teeth. *Marketing Implant Dentistry* offers different internal marketing approaches, which can be utilized by doctors to bring more implant patients to their practices and increase case acceptance.

Described methodologies related to running an implant study club can be used by surgical specialists to expand the size of their existing implant practices in an effective and consistent manner.

I'm very excited about *Marketing Implant Dentistry* by Marcus Hines. I fully believe that the implant practice marketing model described in this book will help fellow practitioners to take their implant practices to the next level, resulting in more patients benefiting from this invaluable service, a more fulfilling professional lifestyle, and the financial success that comes along with it.

Hamid R. Shafie, DDS CAGS
Director of Postdoctoral Implant Training
Department of Oral and Maxillofacial Surgery
Washington Hospital Center
President/Chief Knowledge Officer
American Institute of Implant Dentistry

Introduction

For more than 12 years I have worked in implant dentistry as a sales representative, followed by my current position where I serve as Director of Full Arch Solutions for a major dental implant company. Early on, never in my deepest thoughts did I believe a segment of dentistry was capable of retaining my interest as much as this niche has. I am intrigued by a lot of things, but I'm not sure anything else will ever interest me enough to sit down and write a marketing book about it.

Eventually, I recognized a very large void between what doctors understand clinically with respect to implant dentistry and best practices in attracting and influencing patients to accept a dental implant treatment plan. Consequently, far less patients are benefiting from dental implants compared to what is possible.

Early on, I often found this discipline to be very perplexing, so much so that I almost left the field of dentistry all together. No matter how much I tried, I could not understand how an invaluable service, so capable of helping an immeasurable amount of people, only benefits a relative few.

When I first began selling dental implants, like many dental professionals, I was led to believe that the reason most people chose to replace their missing teeth with traditional crown and bridge was mostly because they can't afford dental implants. "Implants are too expensive," "Insurance doesn't cover implants," or "My patients can't afford implants" is the frame of reference many doctors and their staff members continue to operate from. And for some time I, too, bought into this notion.

Once I began to witness the most unsuspecting offices, usually located in lower- to median-income areas, perform far more dental implant procedures than some offices located in the more affluent areas, I could never again be brainwashed into believing the average patient could not afford implant dentistry. And like a lightning bolt, I suddenly understood that offices performing well above average implant numbers generally take a systematic approach toward marketing and patient communications, while offices that merely dabble in implant dentistry generally believe there is no significant benefit over traditional crown and bridge or believe they are held hostage by dental insurance and have a patient base that has limited financial resources.

I was also frequently baffled by the amount of resources the more advanced clinicians spent on clinical training compared to the resources these same doctors apply toward internal marketing. It's not that I believe doctors spend too much on training. In fact, if you ask me, the average doctor doesn't take nearly as much hands-on dental implant-related continuing education as they should. But since no dental implant procedure can be performed until and unless the patient agrees to a proposed treatment plan, it behooves the clinician and staff to increase the amount of resources applied toward marketing the services of implant dentistry within their practice.

Dr. Kian Djawdan of Annapolis, MD, is an example of a clinician who makes considerable investments in both his clinical skill set and dental implant-marketing efforts. Having earned diplomate status in both the ABOI and ICOI, Dr. Djawdan knows you don't experience long-term success in consistently attracting new full-arch implant patients, as well as achieve high levels of case acceptance, without a meaningful investment in marketing. Dr. Michael Tischler of Woodstock, NY, is another example of a well-trained clinician who understands how to market their implant practice.

But some of the most superiorly trained implant clinicians don't always understand how to best inform a patient of the implant treatment they need, nor do they know how to ask the patient to move forward with treatment with authority. This results in so many of their patients never being given a fair chance to say "yes" to a well-thought-out dental implant treatment plan.

Attracting a steady stream of dental implant patients to your practice requires taking a systematic approach. And influencing patients to accept your dental implant treatment plan has a heck of a lot more to do with understanding who is sitting on the opposite side of the table and what it will take to have your recommendations resonate with that individual. Significant focus on case presentation, visual aids, verbal skills, patient education, staff training, networking, and the like goes hand in hand with clinical training when it comes to being a top performer in implant dentistry.

Be compelling

There is a very popular ABC acronym in sales that stands for "Always Be Closing." I often repurpose this acronym in dentistry to represent "Always Be Compelling." I am thoroughly convinced that if you are compelling in the delivery of your recommendations, you can help as many people as you would like to help with dental implants. However, merely suggest dental implants as an alternative to traditional crown and bridge, and your influence over the patient's decision will be as good as dead. The average patient wants to be led by you. When doctors and their staff members are compelling in the delivery of their implant recommendations, more often than not, ultimately the patient accepts the recommendations.

To an even greater degree, clinicians that perform the most full-arch dental implant procedures usually understand the enormous influence they can have over the patient who is missing most or all of their teeth. Their case presentations are generally well thought out and spoken in layman terms, and they use great visual aids to help the patient appreciate what is possible through implant dentistry.

Washington, D.C.-based prosthodontist Dr. Hamid Shafie has authored two clinical books on implant dentistry and lectures around the world on full-arch immediate occlusal loading. In his professional lectures, he is obviously expected to speak in the most technical of terms. But set him in front of a patient in need of implants, and all these technical terms get tossed out the window. In my observation of his patient communications, to say he's compelling may be a bit of an understatement. I haven't seen anyone more capable of encouraging a patient to accept a full-arch, fixed implant-supported prosthesis. Dr. Shafie's ability to simplify his discussion of implant dentistry only requires the patient to have about a fifth-grade education to understand that it makes sense to act on his advice.

If you are pleased with your clinical skill set but lack the marketing expertise to attract and influence potential implant patients to move forward with treatment, this book was written with you in mind. But understand that becoming a better marketer of dental implant services will most likely require you to see the implant world differently than you presently do. If you attempt to manage your marketing mindset solely through the lens of a clinician who still has most or all of their natural teeth, chances are you will fail to grow your implant business to your satisfaction. Growing your implant business requires you to be capable of managing your marketing efforts through the oral health realities of your patients, not your own.

Rest assured that I have no intention of ever attempting to instruct you on anything clinical. I studied marketing and sales in college, not dentistry. But if you will open your mind enough to heed my dental implant marketing advice and actually follow through by taking action, over the course of the next 12- to 24- to 36-month period, you will position yourself to perform far more dental implant procedures than you did over the same time frames in the past.

The notion that your patients can't afford your dental implant services should never be allowed to dominate your mindset, nor should you or your staff members speak such discouraging words. This is regardless of how intimidating the fees may seem or what you think the patient can afford. On the heartfelt advice of the dental professional, so frequently it's the most unassuming patients that are willing to follow through with the most sophisticated and costly dental implant treatment plans. If you have been in business long enough, you have no doubt had this experience in other areas of your practice.

By the way, being compelling is not just about performing more dental implant procedures—it is a very powerful universal principle that can help you to get what you want out of life. The late motivational speaker Zig Ziglar used to say, "You can have everything in life you want, if you will help enough other people get what they want." When you are compelling, you inspire people to want more, to take action, to do something, and to be inspired. In fact, being compelling is how I ultimately got to meet my all-time favorite musician.

How I met my all-time favorite musician

I would like to share a personal story with you here, only because I believe there is great value in examples of how the universe conspires around you and others when you have a definite chief aim. This experience is also fitting to my underlying message in this book.

I grew up in Detroit, MI, in the 1970s and 1980s, and so I have always been partial to American-made cars and Motown music—Marvin Gay, Diana Ross and the Supremes, The Jackson 5, Temptations, and Commodores (featuring Lionel Richie). I could go on. But my all-time favorite musician has always been Stevie Wonder. He is a musical genius. Elton John once said of Stevie Wonder's *Songs in the Key of Life* album, "For me, it's the best album ever made, and I'm always left in awe after I listen to it."

Back in June of 2012, my siblings and I were discussing the fact that our dad would celebrate his 90th birthday in January of 2013. So we decided to give him a big birthday bash and invite family and close friends to share in our celebration of him. As we drew up the guest list, my brother Fred said, "I'm not sure how we can ever make it happen, but it would be great if we were to somehow have Stevie Wonder attend dad's party."

Instantly, my siblings and I appreciated Fred's idea because we all knew that before he was dubbed "Little Stevie Wonder," he grew up around the corner from my father's Hines Bros. Auto Repair shop on the west side of Detroit. My dad told stories of how Stevie Wonder and his brother and friends would often play around his repair shop. He'd give them pocket change and encourage Stevie Wonder to use his singing talents for good. But that was back in the 1950s when he was a kid. Now, some six decades later, we're talking about the 25 Grammy Award-winning, 100 million album/singles-selling, Martin Luther King Jr. holiday-inspiring, worldly beloved figure, and philanthropist Stevie Wonder! How the heck do we pull this one off?

At the time that Fred made this suggestion, he was unaware of the resources I had. You see, it suddenly dawned on me that I had never mentioned to any of my siblings that my wife Sandra and I share a close mutual friend with Stevie Wonder. This mutual friend is such a dear acquaintance of his that just 2 years prior, Sandra and I watched Stevie Wonder sing at her wedding.

So naturally I offered to handle the process of inviting Mr. Wonder to the birthday party since I stood the best chance of getting an invite in front of him. I suppose that I could have simply handed over an invitation, but I proceeded to put together a letter outlining how my dad is a retired army veteran who fought in WWII, was married to my late mother, Fay Hines, for 60 years and to their union raised 14 children. I also reminded Mr. Wonder of my father's business that he frequented as a child, and I mentioned the fact that my father was proud to have been a positive influence on him and other children in that neighborhood. I even cited a reference to my father that Mr. Wonder had made during a nationally televised interview with Tavis Smiley in 2010.

Once I was done making my case in a well-thought-out and *compelling* letter, I handed over a copy to our mutual friend and asked if she would see to it that he receives it. She agreed to make it happen and said, "He'll be in town in two weeks. I will read your letter to Stevie myself."

Not only did Stevie Wonder attend, but to about 120 family members and close friends, he modestly shared some very kind, reminiscent words about my dad. He then followed his comments by singing his famous rendition of "Happy Birthday" and another one of his famous hits. How cool is that?!

Was I conscious of the possibility of being told "no?" Of course I was. But if being denied included the fact that I was compassionate and compelling in my efforts, I could have found solace in simply knowing that Mr. Wonder understands why my siblings and I believe our father is a living legend.

Fortunately, Mr. Wonder was as excited to be back in the presence of my father and some of my older cousins, as we were to have him. I had no way of knowing this until he arrived. Why else would he go through the trouble of fitting this occasion in between a South American benefit concert the week before and a presidential inauguration appearance the following week? When I greeted him at the door, the first thing he asked was if Ricky, my first cousin, was present. And by the time the party was nearing its end, it was evident to his bodyguard that Mr. Wonder has great respect for my father. He suggested that it's rare when he sticks around to chat and take photos for as long as he did.

Here is the point I want to make. So often, the most difficult part of any worthwhile intention is simply coming up with the idea itself. Once my brother Fred established the vision, without understanding my resources, only then could everything else begin to take its course, and I could do my part to put together a compelling request.

Only you can establish the vision for your patient

Your patients depend on you to establish the vision. When you establish the vision for your prospective implant patient and make a compelling case that inspires that patient to want to agree with you, you immediately increase the chances that the patient will agree to your dental implant treatment plan. And when you are compelling, there is no way of knowing what your patient will say "yes" to.

In my case, I was able to facilitate a priceless desire for both my family and for Mr. Wonder. Unless you make a compelling case for implant dentistry to the larger percentage of your patients with missing teeth, you may never experience the feeling of euphoria that other clinicians routinely experience by knowing that only they could facilitate the priceless desire for another individual to regain basic oral functionality or to prevent long-term catastrophes that the average patient has no way of anticipating.

So many of your patients with missing teeth just want an opportunity to smile again with confidence. So many denture-wearing patients just want the ability to publically eat corn on the cob and to enjoy a flavorful medium-rare porterhouse steak again without having to lace their gums with glue and swallow large chunks of meat. Some of your partial-denture-wearing patients are simply sick with the embarrassment they face each evening after placing their teeth in a cup before kissing their newlywed good-night. Others just want to have a prosthesis that no longer look like horse teeth and will move mountains to replace an eight-year-old bridge that they never really liked in the first place.

Finally, some patients just want the best that healthcare has to offer and will readily pay a premium to have a single tooth replaced with a dental implant once the facts are understood. And that same patient may ultimately hold you accountable, in retrospect, if they believe their healthcare has suffered because the proper "Informed Consent" was not given.

You can't possibly know what will motivate each patient to accept your dental implant treatment plan. Furthermore, you have no idea what they can afford, what resources they have, or to what extent they will go through to smile, eat, and spare the embarrassment. Yet, if your patient is generally pleased with your services, you may be his or her only opportunity to gain exposure to a dental implant-based solution to their problem since they are not actively seeking a new dental care home.

With each patient, you can make a compelling case for their implant treatment plan. If your case is compelling enough, you will soon discover the deeply embedded reasons that motivate patients to accept $5,000, $25,000, or $50,000+ dental implant treatment plans. The good news is that implant dentistry is such an amazing service that it's really not very difficult to deliver a compelling story. Be compelling and your patients will accept your treatment plans in larger numbers.

It is my sincere hope that as you read this book, you will discover multiple approaches to attracting dental implant patients to your practice and multiple approaches for influencing patients to accept your proposed dental implant treatment plans. For me, *Marketing Implant Dentistry* has been a labor of love. Nothing would please me more about this effort than to know that more of your patients are experiencing the benefits of implant dentistry, in part due to one or more pearls you picked up from my book. Best of luck to you!

CHAPTER 1

Visual aids and verbal skills

Successfully explaining the true benefits of dental implants to the layman patient is no easy task. Using models, animations, and the proper verbal skills to get your point across is a very effective way to make an otherwise complicated process easy to understand by the masses.

Most people are unfamiliar with the true benefits of dental implants. And since we all are layman in some form or fashion, we benefit anytime uncharted territory is explained in a way that helps us to "get it." News channels use models and animations all the time to make their more complicated stories easily digestible.

For instance, when the US Navy SEALS raided Bin Laden's Pakistan compound, killed him, and captured his body, helmet cams were worn by the two-dozen members of SEAL Team Six to stream this undertaking back to the White House where the president and other dignitaries witnessed it in real time. The raid was reported to have taken somewhere around 40 minutes, but what you and I and the rest of the general public were privy to through the various news outlets, including a *60 Minutes* interview of a SEAL Team Six member, was a tabletop-sized replica of Bin Laden's massive compound structure and a very short, dumbed-down reenactment of this event through animated video. Using a model of Bin Laden's compound, this Navy SEAL member walked us through the process they had experienced in taking out the world's most wanted individual. And by the end of

Marketing Implant Dentistry: Attract and Influence Patients to Accept Your Dental Implant Treatment Plan, First Edition. Marcus Hines.
© 2016 John Wiley & Sons, Inc. Published 2016 by John Wiley & Sons, Inc.

this short interview, you felt like you had a pretty good understanding of exactly how this complicated mission was executed.

Physicians make great use of visual aids

Physicians who are routinely required to treat their patients by incorporating surgery tend to use visual aids to explain the clinical rationale, far more frequently than dental professionals do. CNN's chief medical correspondent, Dr. Sanjay Gupta, a neurosurgeon, uses skull and brain models coupled with animations all the time to describe how different areas of the brain function, the effects of traumatic brain injuries, and the rationale of various brain surgeries. The host of *The Dr. Oz Show*, Dr. Mehmet Oz, a cardiothoracic surgeon, uses animations, models, and props routinely to help communicate various medical conditions and the rationale for the required surgical treatment to his television viewers.

Developing illustrations, models, and animations to describe a sophisticated event or process like implant dentistry requires training and creativity. So imagine what it would cost to produce lifelike jaw and dental implant models for only your office. Now, add this cost to the expense of producing animated videos for use in only your office, say, to demonstrate how a sinus expands following tooth loss or to describe the process of bone resorption, bone grafting with the aid of tenting screws, and dental implant placements and restorations.

Any idea of the required time and resources necessary to get it just right for these and 200 plus other clinical scenarios to be turned into animated videos? Fortunately, since video animations have already been produced and are sold on a massive scale for a relatively small fee, you don't have to go through this effort to dramatically enhance communications between your office and your prospective dental implant patients. Relative to the value of these tools the investment is miniscule. Good visual aids is one of the best internal marketing investments any dental implant provider can make.

Better to show empathy, not sympathy

Like good use of visual aids, making the best use of your verbal skills when presenting your implant treatment plans will pay dividends in case acceptance. Numerous leaders in case presentation technique have suggested that you must first *listen* to the patient and develop a good understanding of what their desires are before attempting to present your recommendations. In other words, empathize. I could not agree more with this notion. In any sales situation, the empathetic listener will come out on top far more frequently than the individual who is only concerned with getting their point across about their product or service.

Where I differ is when some of the same authorities suggest, for example, that if the otherwise healthy 70-year-old, partial-denture wearer wants to replace her removable prosthesis because it no longer looks good or functions well, it does little good to broach the subject of dental implants when her primary financial goal is to maximize her insurance benefits and pay as little out of pocket as possible. I disagree wholeheartedly with this view when it comes to dental implants. And in its truest sense, because dental implants may be such a patient's only hope of having her desired functionality restored, this approach does not necessarily show empathy. If anything, this is sympathy, and being sympathetic should be left to family and friends.

If it is safe to assume you chose to read this book because you believe that more patients will benefit when you perform more dental implant procedures, then you must become comfortable with exploring all viable solutions with such patients, finances notwithstanding. Showing empathy requires more effort than sympathy. When you are compassionately empathetic, your strong desire to help the patient forces you to express the best solutions to their problems. Sympathy allows you to merely feel bad for the patient and does not necessarily require offering a viable solution for whatever reason.

Replacing an ill-fitting partial denture with implants for the 70-year-old lady is not the same as proposing a $20,000 laminate veneer case for a 60-year-old woman who has shown no interest in esthetics or a $5,000 orthodontic case for a 35-year-old male who presents with a diastema between his maxillary central incisors but has otherwise healthy and well-functioning teeth. The same patient might have made it clear during the doctor's discovery process that improved esthetics are of no concern to him and that he prefers this gap, as it represents his identity and family trait. Therefore, you proceed to present only what is necessary to keep this patient healthy and happy. This is empathy.

But to refuse to bring up dental implants to a healthy 70-year-old patient because you think she's too old or you fear appearing as though you are taking advantage of a little old lady is an expression of sympathy not empathy. Moreover such patients are robbed of their right to understand dental implants as a viable option. In my opinion, this belongs in the same category of neglect with the dentist or hygienist who agrees to provide a routine prophylaxis to the advanced periodontally diseased patient without discussing the fact that the long-term solution may involve more costly surgical procedures.

Implants are worth more than replacing missing teeth

The literature proves time and again that implants help to prevent jawbone atrophy, positively affect muscle tone, and promote the patient's ability to chew and grind all types of foods superiorly. Whether the patient accepts or refuses a certain treatment option is irrelevant. What is important is that the dental professional discloses the treatment options to the patient—including implants—in a way that the patient is best capable of sorting out their options. The onus is then placed on the patient to accept or deny the recommended treatment.

Dr. Roger P. Levin, president and CEO of the Levin Group, Inc. says, "Although not every patient needs implants right now, every single patient should be made aware of implants. Therefore, dentists have an obligation to educate all patients about this treatment option. Avoid screening patients based on your perception of *their* interest level or ability to pay" (Levin, 2011a).

Whether the ideal implant treatment plan will cost the 70-year-old patient $5,000 or $50,000, that patient deserves to understand her options for having missing teeth replaced with dental implants as much as any patient who is much younger. There are no two ways about it.

Everything begins with asking the right questions

In his *New York Times* Best Seller, *The 7 Habits of Highly Effective People*, Dr. Stephen R. Covey's fifth habit is "Seek First to Understand, Then to Be Understood." The title of this habit says everything you need to know about it. Dr. Covey explains, "The essence of empathic listening is not that you agree with someone; it's that you fully, deeply, understand that person, emotionally as well as intellectually" (Covey, 1989).

Before you begin to put together any dental implant treatment plan, you have to first understand what your patients' present frustrations, dislikes, and limitations are with their current circumstances and also what their motives, desires, and expectations are for the replacement prostheses. For example, perhaps they can no longer chew their food on the right side, or their lower denture has begun to move when they smile, or the bridgework in the front of their mouth causes them to blow air bubbles when they talk. Understanding what the limiting functionality is will go a long way in helping to develop and present an implant treatment plan that resonates. These are all the reasons why patients develop a sense of urgency for replacing their missing teeth or, for that matter, have no sense of urgency and will need your help with creating one.

Maybe the patient's daughter is going to be married in 6 months, her flexible spending account will expire in 60 days, or your patient has recently suffered a heart attack and his registered dietitian has placed him on a heart-healthy diet that includes nuts rich in omega-3 fatty acids and mono- and polyunsaturated fats like walnuts, almonds, and macadamia nuts. Such a patient most likely will find it difficult to chew the recommended raw, leafy green salads as well.

As you know, often your patients will volunteer much of this information, and other times you will have to help them share. The best way to have your patients acknowledge their limiting functionalities, motives, and hot buttons is to ask good questions before and during your clinical evaluation. Box 1.1 is an example of the types of questions that should be asked. Don't worry about the fact that some questions will cause you to "lead your witness." You are a dentist, not a lawyer, so no one will stand up and object. Besides, if you ask the questions the right way, your patients won't even suspect that you are gathering details that will later help you to influence them to replace their missing teeth with dental implants.

Box 1.1 Before the dentist can be effective at presenting a treatment plan that speaks to the patient's concerns, he/she must first use questions designed to uncover the patient's issues.

Ask the right questions

1 How long have you had your current bridge?
2 What do you like about your partial denture, if anything?
3 Are you able to chew your food very well with your denture in place?
4 Do you like the way your denture looks?
5 Have any of your personal relationships given you any feedback—good, bad, or indifferent—about your teeth?
6 Are you forced to wear denture glue to stabilize your denture? If so, what happens if you don't wear denture glue?
7 Do you have any short deadlines that you need your new teeth by? If so, what are the reasons?
8 Is it difficult to clean around your bridgework?
9 Does food seem to get trapped around your bridge?
10 Do you find it more convenient to eat with or without your denture in place?
11 Are you self-conscious, in any way, about eating out in public or in social gatherings with friends and family members?
12 Do you understand why tooth loss leads to jawbone loss?
13 Do you like the way your smile looks with your partial denture in place?
14 Do you mind taking your partial denture in and out to clean it, or would you prefer that it doesn't have to be removed, like natural teeth?
15 Do you routinely suffer from heartburn?
16 Are you presently taking medication for acid reflux disease?
17 What do you miss most about not having good teeth?
18 Are you able to routinely enjoy foods like apples, corn on the cob, or nuts?
19 How long would you like to see your next set of teeth last you before they no longer function well?
20 What would make you happiest about your teeth?

The power of visual aids

As much as dental professionals insist on visual aids and good communications from sales representatives to become familiar with products they show interest in—such as equipment, handpieces, or dental software—so often doctors expect the patient to understand the rationale of receiving, say, a sinus lift, a bone or soft tissue graft, or a dental

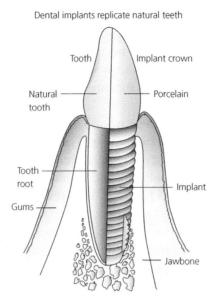

Dental implants replicate natural teeth

Tooth

Implant crown

Natural tooth

Porcelain

Tooth root

Implant

Gums

Jawbone

Figure 1.1 Show the patients what an implant looks like compared to a natural tooth.

implant, all without the use of the proper visual aids. This results in having to follow a path of least resistance. It's no wonder why practitioners agree to some PPOs that require discounting fees down to next to nothing or find themselves held hostage by the limiting confines of a patient's $1,000 insurance maximum. It is very difficult to convince someone to pay top dollar for something they don't understand.

Imagine for a moment a knowledgeable and experienced dental implant sales representative shows up at your office for a scheduled meeting. The representative's goal is to sell you his implant system. There's just one problem; he was never given a surgical kit to detail his advanced or premium user-friendly system. He has no oversized replica of his premium implant to show you why his system is superior to the more familiar and lower-priced implant system you have been using for years. You might wonder why he even bothered to show up. Can you imagine buying this implant system without having the ability to play with a lifelike model or to put your hands on a surgical kit? Of course you can't, especially at a premium price. The patient needs to see an implant in relation to a tooth (as in Figure 1.1) and to be given a thorough explanation of its benefits.

You could learn a lesson from my contractor

When the intent is to persuade your patients to agree to an elective procedure that is perceived to be the most expensive option, then you must do what other professions who sell an expensive product or service do. Use solid visual aids that are more persuasive than anything you can say.

When my wife Sandra and I were planning to build a deck for our house, we were particular about how we wanted this deck to be. We met with two companies. The first company is well known in the Washington, D.C., region for building quality fences, windows, doors, and decks. This company had built a fence for us at our previous home that we happened to be pleased with it. They also had built a neighbor's deck that we liked. The salesman came out and asked questions, took some measurements, showed us table samples, and talked to us for about an hour at the kitchen table, and I suppose he was off to meet another prospect.

The second company was smaller but came highly recommended from an oral surgeon and implant customer, Dr. Sharon Russell. Dr. Russell and her husband, Mark, had used this company and were quite pleased with Kirk, the owner, and his team's ability to execute.

Kirk took measurements and brought table samples as well, but before he started, he said, "By the time I leave you today, if nothing else, my goal is to educate you and to have you fully understand everything you need to know about what a good quality deck represents and what different options are available to you." As a salesman who shares this philosophy, I was now all ears. After asking multiple questions and speaking with us at the table for an hour or so, he took us out to his oversized, double-wide cargo truck, which was literally like a showroom on wheels. You go inside this truck, and Kirk's got about six different decking materials in all types of different colors and built-in countertops, allowing him to demonstrate side by side why brand A is better than B and why brand C is even better than A. How's that for visual aids?

He'd go on to demonstrate different types of guardrails that were available, including lighting that could be added to the rails and steps to really give it a classy look during those summer nights while playing host to a few guests. Four hours later, when Kirk had answered all of our questions and finished educating us on the value of composite materials compared to treated wood and taking all types of measurements and it was time to go, we'd pretty much decided that he was our guy.

We felt like we had seen all the samples and had each of our questions answered and that he had enough expertise to give us exactly what we were looking for. Was he more expensive? Yes, pound for pound, the deck alone was slightly more expensive. But because he offered so much more of a vision and gave us more expert-opinionated options to consider compared to the other company, we also agreed to have him do much more than just build a deck. Kirk also helped us make an informed decision about the advantages of having a stamped concrete patio beneath the deck and a paved walkway alongside the house, which would be constructed at the same time as the deck. As it turned out, we spent significantly more money with Kirk because we opted to have him perform a more comprehensive project compared to simply having a deck built, which is the only thing the first company presented.

Here's another point worth making: Kirk's deck required us to dig deeper into our resources, and from the questions he posed to the compelling visual aids he used to demonstrate his recommendations, he helped paint an imaginary picture that inspired us to feel like we could never go back to only wanting a simple deck. This is good salesmanship.

I took time to tell this story because whether it's selling a deck or a treatment plan for a torn rotator cuff, knee replacement, or dental implants, the proposal or treatment plan must be defined in the most layman, understandable terms possible—verbally and visually. When it comes to making your case for replacing missing teeth with dental implants, there is no substitute for good *visual aids* and *verbal skills* that inspire people to take action. Inadequate verbal skills result in otherwise great treatment plans being turned down, time and again.

How much time did you spend understanding the patient's desires? By the time the patient leaves your office, how well educated are they about the multiple advantages of replacing missing teeth with dental implants? How descriptive were you in sharing the benefits behind your implant solutions? How influential are your visual aids to someone that knows little to nothing about implant dentistry? Educating your patient is paramount.

Do you have the fortitude to say to your patient "No matter what method of tooth replacement you choose, you will be well educated on your options"?

What I wouldn't do to have a penny for every time I hear a dentist say, "I'd like to do more dental implants, but my patients can't afford them." So many patients deny your dental implant treatment proposition for no good reason except that they don't understand what you are proposing, at least not enough to say "yes" to your $4,000 or $40,000 implant treatment plan.

Your patients aren't broke, but your delivery may be broken

If you're not using the proper verbal skills and taking advantage of all the visual aids that are available to help you educate your patients and make your case, it's costing you in discounted fees and lost caseload. I might have called this chapter "Sell more dental implant services," but in my experience, most dentists don't like to see themselves as "selling." Please don't confuse the issue; this chapter is all about internal marketing, selling yourself and selling your dental implant services. There is no way around it.

Here's the reality. Because a patient tells you "I don't have the money" doesn't necessarily mean the patient can't afford what you are offering. The more complex the case, the higher the fees, and the less your patients understand you. This results in less acceptance of your proposed treatment plans, lost production, and lack of treatment received by the patient. People will spend money on what they want, but not necessarily on what they need. The challenge you face is having the patient have a strong enough *want* for the very services they *need*.

In the book *Beyond Selling*, authors Dan S. Bagley III and Edward J. Reese tell an old Las Vegas joke about a stressed, agitated, and unshaved businessman who approaches a stranger outside one of the casinos and begs, "Could you please spare me a few extra dollars?" The needy gentleman goes on to state, "My wife and kids are with me, and we don't have any money for food or for a place to stay. Any amount will help. Please!" The stranger responds by asking, "If I were to give you some money, how do I know that you won't take the money and go inside and gamble it away?" The distraught man looked at the stranger indignantly, pulled out a wad of twenties, and exclaimed, "Gambling money I've got!" (Bagley, III & Reese, 1988).

The authors go on to explain that in nearly all selling situations, there is money for what is wanted badly enough. Most of the time, when a customer professes to lack the money to purchase a product or service, the situation can be translated to mean, "I am not yet ready to trade my big sack of money for that little stack of potential value that you have demonstrated so far."

The same patient who tells you they can't afford to replace three missing teeth with dental implants will leave your office and go pay cash for a wide-screen, flat-panel supersmart television that they have had an eye on for months. It happens all the time. Why? It's usually because not enough has been done to help this patient desire replacing his three missing teeth with dental implants as much as he desires to replace his 3-year-old, flat-panel television with the newer, bigger, smarter version he enjoyed watching at his friend's Super Bowl party.

Verbal skills

Kirk (from the deck/patio scenario) started out by verbalizing his mission to my wife and I. Almost immediately, he stated, "If nothing else, my goal is to educate you…." In other words, even if you choose to do nothing at all or you opt for a lower-cost solution or even decide to use my competitor, at minimum, you will gain value from this discussion, guaranteed. That's priceless!

Let's consider verbal skills for a moment. I have sat in on numerous implant case presentations given to the patient by the dentist or a staff member, and though not always, but usually, when the patient refuses the dental implant treatment plan, it has something to do with the fact that the mission was not to thoroughly educate the patient first. If this were the case, just like Kirk, doctors would prepare their scripts in a way that touches the very essence of that patient's soul by giving them a message that resonates.

I recall one in particular like it was yesterday. I had been coaching this dentist on exactly what to say in this specific case. He asked me to observe and give feedback. I immediately noticed the only visual aid he had was the patient's panoramic X-ray. He had not followed through on my advice to purchase implant models. The presentation was similar to Discussion Example 1.1.

Discussion example 1.1

Doctor   Mrs. Jones, I have put together a treatment plan for you to replace your missing tooth [in the back of your mouth]. Traditionally, we would cut down your two adjacent teeth and give you a fixed bridge just like the one you have on the other side of your mouth, but today, a better approach is to place a dental implant under your gums and have it serve as the anchor for the crown.

Patient   But I haven't had any problems with my bridgework. It feels just like my regular teeth. Why wouldn't you just do another bridge?

Doctor   To do a bridge, I would have to cut down two perfectly good teeth in order to give you a bridge, and this can potentially shorten the life span of the two teeth we cut down. The other problem with this method is that once we take out a tooth, you begin to lose bone in that area unless we replace the removed tooth with a dental implant.

Patient   Well, how much will this implant cost me compared to the bridge?

Doctor   Actually, the bridge and the implant are about the same cost—$3,600 for the bridge and $3,800 for an implant. I had Sharon check with your insurance company, and your insurance company won't cover any cost associated with the implant surgery. They will pay 50% for the cost of your implant crown or 50% of the total cost of the bridge- work. All told, the implant will cost you about a $1,000 more out of pocket.

Patient   Well to be honest with you Dr. Jackson, I'm in sales, and it's been a very slow year, and I can't afford to pay anymore [out of pocket] than is necessary. I think we should just go with the bridge. After all, I pay good money for that insurance, and I'd like to be able to take advantage of it.

Doctor   OK Mrs. Jones, then we'll have Sharon get you scheduled for your next [bridgework] appointment.

Immediately following his presentation to the patient, he said to me, "See, I told you; if these insurance companies would just pay more for implant treatment [surgery], I would perform more dental implant procedures." He said this as if it were the insurance com- panies' fault that patients deny implant treatment.

Please understand that no one can ever accuse me of being an apologist for insurance companies. I think "dental insurance" is a mis- nomer. What other business can totally ignore the rising cost of infla- tion for decades by offering the same old lousy $1,000–$1,500 yearly maximum benefit while consistently raising premiums and get away with it like dental insurance companies do? But never is it an insur- ance company's fault if the patient refuses treatment, especially if you have not been effective in your communications.

This dentist's verbal communications were inadequate. That said, it wasn't inadequate verbal skills alone or even dental insurance that cost him this implant case. After all, his presentation included the neg- atives of "cutting down the teeth" and the ill effects of "bone loss" in the absence of a tooth root. What he did not do is *show* (visual aids) the patient everything he was *telling* (verbal skills) her, and in so doing, he failed to have his patient understand everything she needed to know to make an informed decision. You can't be effective by showing a panoramic X-ray if the patient doesn't know what she is looking at.

This was an attractive, well-dressed, middle-aged woman who clearly cared deeply about her outward appearance. She was also fit and trim, which would indicate she cared about her health. She might as well have held a sign that said, "Look at me, aren't I beautiful?" Because this dentist's presentation involved no three-dimensional visual aids such as a dental implant model to demonstrate to her dominant visual senses, well, I'm guessing she probably retained less than 10% of what he had to say. Even though she has a bridge, she's never seen what it looks like to have her teeth cut down, and she certainly can't appreciate what buccal bone loss looks like on a dark and hard-to-read, two-dimensional, panoramic X-ray.

If you are not using dental implant models and animated software to help deliver your presentation, you are doing this the hard way, and you are most likely receiving the aforementioned patient response far more than necessary. Today's current implant models and animations are so good that choosing not to use them is sort of like taking a 1-hour, 3-mile brisk walk to your office every day in 90° temperatures when you can simply get in the car, turn up the AC, and be there in 8 minutes.

Contrast *Discussion example* 1.1 with *Discussion example* 1.2. Understand that these are real differences that can be quantified. The combination of inadequate verbal skills and lack of solid visual aids was not enough to influence the patient to accept the recommended dental implant treatment in Example 1.1. Yet the solid verbal skills and the indisputable models clearly made the difference in having the patient accept the implant option over the bridge in Example 1.2.

Work out the financials

The only thing left for your office manager to do now is to find a reasonable way to collect the patient's balance. If the patient has decent credit, perhaps, she will consider applying for one of the healthcare-specific credit cards. These companies will usually offer a 12-month, interest-free option to the patient and take a higher discount from you, the provider, on the back end. If this is not an option, maybe the patient is willing to pay for half the procedure

Discussion example 1.2

The conversation should have carried on something like this.

Doctor   Mrs. Jones, I understand that your cash flow may be an issue, and if I were you, at face value, I'd probably think going with the bridge would save me the most money, too. Most patients do, but it's actually the opposite; it's the bridge that will cost you far more than the implant, every time.

Patient   Oh really? How's that so, since my insurance will pay more for the bridge?

Doctor   It's simple; in my experience, you can expect the bridge to last you only about 10, maybe 15 years if you're lucky. Long term, the bridge will cost you much more because it is very unnatural to chop down these two perfectly fine, adjacent teeth to small nubs [demonstrating on the bridge vs. implant model; see Figure 1.2]. It's also very unnatural to then lock the two adjacent teeth together to form a "bridge." Can you see how difficult it would be to keep the areas between these two teeth clean?

Patient   I guess I never thought about that. But aren't there brushes available to clean those areas?

Doctor   Yes, and if you were to ask me how many of my patients use them effectively, I would have to tell you a very small percentage, which leads me to the next point. In roughly 10 years, more or less, when the bridge fails, it's not uncommon that one of these adjacent teeth [demonstrating on the bridge vs. implant model] will either need a root canal or will need to be removed because of decay. If one of these teeth has to

Implant and three-unit bridge

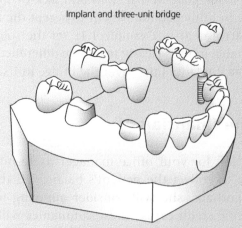

Figure 1.2   The implant and three-unit bridge model is a must-have.

be removed, at that point we will need to aggressively chop down this next one or two teeth, strip them of their enamel, and make an even longer bridge. If a three-unit bridge cost you $3,600 today, at best, a bigger, four-unit bridge will most certainly cost you $7,000 in 10 years, at minimum. Your maximum dental benefit will still only be $1,000, which means you will be forced to pay $6000 out of pocket for your second bridge. Both bridges combined, your total cost will be well over $10,000; and for many people, this is a vicious cycle that never ends until they lose all of their teeth. If you're trying to save money, bridgework is not the way to go.

Patient	If I get the implant instead, how long can I expect it to last?
Doctor	You will still be required to keep the implant tooth clean, but an implant tooth is easier to keep clean and does not decay. I now have multiple patients with 20- and 30-plus-year-old dental implants. I can't think of one patient with a 30-year-old bridge. Not only will the implant save you money, as I mentioned before; it will help preserve your jawbone.
Patient	OK, I get it. I see why I have been coming to you for years. No one ever takes the time to explain things to me the way you do.
Doctor	[Laugh] I appreciate your trust more than you know. I'm going to have Lisa come and talk to you about finances. And don't worry, once my surgeon places your implant, it will take about three and a half months before we can deliver your implant crown. Lisa will work out payment terms with you so that by the time the area has healed and you're ready for the crown, you will have had time to satisfy your portion of the implant crown compared to the 2 weeks you would have to satisfy your fees for the bridgework.

with either cash or credit at the time of surgery and the remaining balance just before the crown is delivered.

If neither of these two payment methods is an option, the office manager should explore having the patient pay for the implant services over a 3- to 5-month period, if necessary. This usually works best if you can find an option to secure payment in a way that doesn't require the patient to think about it. In other words, let's assume in the previous scenario that the patient's insurance will pay a net $600 for the implant crown. This will leave the patient with $3,200 out-of-pocket expenses. Your office manager should be prepared to ask, "Would it work if we break down your out-of-pocket expenses into four, equal-monthly payments of $800?" If this is acceptable, the next goal is to secure a form of payment by either scheduled credit card or ACH payment.

If monthly payments can be made with a credit card or ACH, the office manager can create a tickler file that reminds them to secure electronic payment for the agreed-upon amount on the agreed-upon date, over the course of 3–5 months.

All things considered, if you have done a good job at detailing the rationale of receiving a dental implant versus a more traditional alternative, and you give the patient multiple options for covering their costs associated with the implant, far more patients will find a way to pay for the implant therapy you recommend. It is worth noting that you cannot discount the importance of an adequate case presentation when it comes to collecting the fees, no matter how large or small the case. Without a case presentation that resonates with your patient, you will never get to the point of working out payment terms.

Dental implant models

It never made much sense to me that a dentist could spend thousands of dollars on quality implant courses, fly clear across the country in some cases, learn how to provide such a meaningful service, and at the same time, invest little to no effort and resources in the process of demonstrating to patients exactly what a dental implant looks like in the mouth or what the consequences are to the jawbone in the absence of teeth. We want patients to spend $4,500 on an implant to replace a single tooth or $30,000 for an implant-supported, fixed prosthesis, but we choose to appeal to only one of their senses—*auditory*.

In essence, the higher the fee, the more senses you must reach to be effective. Imagine buying a car without first being able to at least see (visual) the available colors, sit inside (touch), and test drive. You might not have to show a patient what a composite filling looks like, but to consistently have patients accept your higher-priced dental implant treatment plans, you had better appeal to their *auditory*, *visual*, and sense of *touch*. Neglect either one of these three senses during your case presentation, and the chances are pretty good that you will lose some implant cases that you would have otherwise closed.

Box 1.2 Some models available for implant case presentations.

Dental implant models

- Implant and three-unit bridge model
- Four-Implant Locator™ abutment lower-overdenture model
- Four-, five-, or six-implant fixed-hybrid model
- Full-arch zirconia bridge model
- Mandible bone-loss model
- Atrophied-ridge mandible model (partially edentulous)
- Perio-defect mandible model
- Three-unit bridge on three-implant model (free end)
- Partial-denture model

A dental implant model is worth its weight in gold, and there is a demonstration model for virtually every type of case you can think of describing to the patient. In my experience, every practitioner should have multiple dental implant models in the consultation room and in each operatory (Box 1.2). Even most of the full-arch, immediate- or delayed-occlusal-loading protocols have their own replica models available. Don't spend $4000 on tuition for the full-arch implant course and sit in the course for 2 days to learn the clinical protocol only to leave the course without the demonstration tools necessary to successfully convince your patients to say, "Yes!" It's being "penny wise and pound foolish" to do so.

Maybe you intend to replace a single tooth and need to demonstrate an implant versus a three-unit bridge as demonstrated in the aforementioned consultation example. There's a model with an *implant* on one side and a *bridge* on the other. Perhaps you intend to demonstrate two options for replacing a denture with four implants supported by Locator® attachments for a removable prosthesis versus four to six implants positioned to support a fixed-hybrid prosthesis (like figures 4.4 and 4.5).

If you're going to be serious about improving your communications with the patient, you need to have several implant models always available to educate your patients. You don't have to purchase them all at once, but know that those most capable of influencing the patient to accept their implant treatment plans usually have, at their disposal, multiple types of models to help the patient appreciate the proposed treatment.

Elevator pitch

According to Wikipedia, an *elevator pitch* is a "short summary ... used to quickly and simply define a person, profession, product, service, organization, or event and its value proposition" (Wikipedia, 2014). The term *elevator pitch* stems from the hypothetical that asks, "What if you found yourself alone in an elevator with the very person that could say yes to your proposition, and before the elevator door opens, you only have a very short period of time to get your point across in the most effective and persuasive way possible? How would you make your pitch?"

Such a pitch must be highly scripted because there is no time to waste. When you are making the case for a dental implant, although not always, but often enough, you will find that your elevator pitch is sufficient to draw strong interest when used in conjunction with good visual aids (Box 1.3).

Dr. Emma Galvan is owner of Dental Seminars, LLC and a full-time practicing dentist. While she does not perform implant surgery, I estimate that each year, Dr. Galvan restores as many implants as any dentist within the upper 10th percentile of implant restorative dentists. Her practice is located in Dundalk, MD, just outside of Baltimore, MD.

Box 1.3 An elevator pitch can be used to introduce the rationale of an implant over bridgework.

Dental implant elevator pitch

Mrs. Smith, unfortunately we can no longer save your tooth, and it needs to come out because of a fractured root. So the question becomes, 'how will we replace it?' Essentially, our two choices are to replace the missing tooth with either a bridge or an implant. The major problem with a bridge is that we have to cut down your two adjacent teeth [demonstrating with a bridge model]. You can also see how the bridge will trap food and cause decay to the two anchoring teeth. When this happens, we have to replace the bridge and eventually remove the decayed teeth that the bridge depends on. This is why a bridge is far more expensive long term. With a dental implant, there is no need to chop down your adjacent teeth [demonstrating with an implant model]. We simply anchor a small screw beneath your gums, and just like the root of a natural tooth, we attach a crown to it, and unlike a bridge, the implant is totally independent of your other teeth. It's that simple. Does that make sense?

Dundalk is a blue-collar, working-class city. I have known Dr. Galvan for several years, and I asked her how she consistently gains case acceptance at such high levels. Here's how she put it:

> Essentially, I have a short script that I've memorized so well that it just flows. I rarely stray away from it, because I know if I stay on course, I stand the best chance of helping the patient make the right decision.

Dr. Galvan may call it a "script," while I refer to it as an "elevator pitch," but essentially, it's one and the same. She can pretty much make this same pitch to any patient needing to replace a missing tooth with an implant, with slight variances.

As impactful as an elevator pitch can be, understand that its intent is not to close the patient on a treatment plan. An effective elevator pitch serves its purpose when it peaks the patients interest just enough to need to know more about what you are proposing. In many instances, it's your staff members who will find themselves in positions to make use of an elevator pitch. Whether it's at the front desk, on the phone, or in the operatory, the staff member capable of delivering an effective elevator pitch can influence a patient in a very positive way.

Could it be that your case presentation just sucks?

Too often, I witness dentists making lackluster presentations of a priceless service like implant dentistry. Yet these same dentists present root canal therapy, post and core, occlusion, orthodontics, third-molar extractions, cosmetic dentistry, periodontal disease, composite fillings, and so on, all with such grace and comprehension. And the patients accept the treatment, in part, because of how well it was presented.

One of my favorite television sitcoms to watch as a teenager was *The Cosby Show* because it was funny, yet there were often lessons to be learned as well. I am reminded of a particular episode when 18-year-old Vanessa went off to college and met a 30-year-old, otherwise respectable man who was already settled into his career, named Dabnis Brickey. While visiting her parents back home, Vanessa used the opportunity to introduce this gentleman to her family for the first time. She would also make it known to her parents that she and Dabnis were engaged to be married and that the two of them had been engaged for 6 months at that point.

Needless to say, the disappointment Vanessa's parents shared for her judgment was obvious. Her father, Dr. Huxtable (played by Bill Cosby), explained it to Dabnis this way: "The fact that we don't like you has nothing to do with your career as a maintenance man. You could be a banker … and we still would not like you." When Dabnis seemed perplexed, Cosby proceeded metaphorically by asking, "What's your favorite food?" Dabnis replied, "Steak." Cosby continued, "Imagine I take the garbage can lid off the can and turn it upside down. I take your nice, juicy Porterhouse steak, potatoes, and sautéed mushrooms, place it on that garbage can lid, and I present it to you. Not too appetizing, is it?" He added, "It's the presentation. That's the way [Vanessa] brought you here; on a garbage can lid."

Cosby's point was obvious. A poor and inadequate presentation will trump great potential every time. It doesn't matter how great of a clinician you are—the presentation is everything. A poor presentation can make an otherwise well-trained and highly experienced clinician appear to be weak and untrustworthy. A great dental implant presentation can make even a mediocre implant clinician appear to be at the top of their game and will help that clinician achieve a high case acceptance rate. If you want to improve your case acceptance in implant dentistry, you must invest in resources that will help you appear at the top of your game in the minds of your prospective dental implant patients.

Implant animations

For as little as about $1000, you can have a complete library of dental animations, including dental implants. There is an animation to demonstrate the advantages of receiving a dental implant with a side-by-side, colorful graphic comparison to the multiple disadvantages of receiving fixed bridgework.

Trust me, no one patient in his or her right mind will opt for a fixed bridge over an implant after viewing some of these animated videos. Remember the dentist I discussed earlier in the chapter who was incapable of convincing his young and attractive patient to receive an implant versus a three-unit bridge? Had he shown her one animation in particular, on top of what he told her, there is no way she would have refused to accept his implant recommendation.

Whatever dental implant procedure you need to convince the patient of, you can do it with the aid of an animation, as demonstrated in Figure 1.3. Sinus lifts, block grafts, bone atrophy, you name it, you can use a well-designed animation to demonstrate virtually any dental implant procedure you can think of. The animation software has become very sophisticated but easy to use. There are several companies that sell dental implant animations, and like anything else, each company attempts to fill a void that the others do not.

Some programs will allow you to personalize your animations. For instance, consider the patient presenting with a failing bridge involving abutment teeth #9 and #11, with a pontic site #10. During the examination, you discover cuspid #11 will require endodontics and a crown. Tooth #10 will require a bone graft and implant placement if the patient accepts your implant treatment plan. Without use of an animation, it is very difficult to have 9 out of 10 patients appreciate what's required for the best results. By enhancing each patient's treatment plan with an

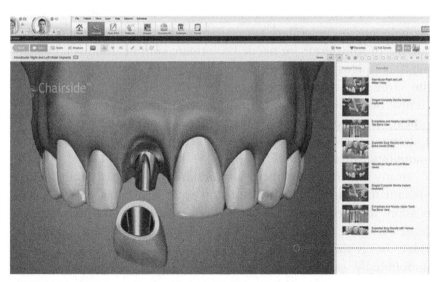

Figure 1.3 In a few seconds, a video animation can make all the difference. Consult-PRO www.consult-PRO.com. Reproduced with permission of Dr. Boris Pulec, CEO Consult-PRO.

animation, you immediately increase your chances of case acceptance 10-fold.

Dr. Justin Moody performs far more dental implants than the average clinician and is an advocate of personalized animated software for dental implant case presentations. In an article titled "Personalize the practice with more digital tools," he explained it this way: "When the program's images and animations are integrated for better understanding, patients not only know what is happening in their mouths, but they feel compelled to do something about it. When patients see what I see, they are empowered to ask questions, and they gain that feeling of co-diagnosis that everyone talks about" (Moody, 2011).

And sometimes a customized animation is most appreciated following the surgical procedure. Often enough, it's the buyer's remorse that makes a patient question your fees, especially if they believe a friend or family member received the same procedure for a lesser fee.

As an implant sales representative, an exceptionally skilled customer shared a patient complaint story with me that had much to do with his patient not understanding why she paid $2875 for her single implant surgery, while her coworker, a patient she referred, more recently paid just $1900 for her single implant surgery. What the complaining patient didn't remember this doctor explaining was that her anterior case required decorticating the buccal wall of her congenitally missing maxillary lateral incisor site, allograft bone material, and use of AlloDerm® for needed soft tissue volume, followed by placing the implant and providing an immediate provisional crown, all in the same visit. The complaining patient spoke very highly of the clinical outcome of her case, but felt slighted when she learned her colleague/friend paid less. In reality, the complaining patient's colleague needed only an implant and required no grafting for the mandibular premolar site.

In my experience, clinicians sometimes forget that patients want implant teeth that look and function well. And most patients can't possibly appreciate what separates one case from another when it comes to costs. In this situation, a customized, 1-minute animated video that is shown postsurgical (if not prior to surgery) would have undoubtedly gone a long ways to help the patient appreciate the unique requirements of her case and stem off any complaints. Such an animated video should also be sent to the restoring doctor in an e-mail to help the dentist understand exactly what treatment took place so that they too can appreciate the surgical fees charged to such a patient.

Leveraging your auxiliary staff for animation demos

As the dentist, you really don't need to spend much of your time in the presence of your patients while they view the animation videos, especially during the treatment planning phase. That's the beauty of an effective animation. It will tell the story for you, in many instances, better than you can tell it yourself.

So train your staff to do it for you. Following the examination, give your staff member some basic background information on what the dental implant case will require, say your good-byes to the patient, and have the implant coordinator queue up the appropriate animation movies to be reviewed by the patient in the consultation room.

No other profession delegates their face-to-face interaction with the patient as well as they do in the medical field. Recently, I went in for my annual physical, and I was not seen by a doctor for either of the two visits. One young lady came and measured my weight, took my blood pressure, and drew blood. I assume she was a registered nurse. When she was done with me, she then sent in a physician's assistant to meet with me, and she asked more questions, followed by intelligible recommendations. I'm sure a doctor was on staff, but for the purposes of my two visits, the auxiliary staff handled my appointment completely.

Certainly, the medical field has its issues, and to some degree, physicians must farm out many of the one-to-one efforts in order to maintain a certain value on their time, but we can learn something from the physicians when it comes to delegating.

Take the time to train your implant coordinator to handle many of the face-to-face interactions that don't necessarily require your presence. This person should reach a point where he or she becomes even more proficient than you will ever be at setting up these videos and reviewing them with patients. You will find that the time it will save you is invaluable.

Summary

It is vital that you approach every potential implant patient with your findings, prognoses, and treatment options. This is your responsibility to the patient. The choice the patient makes with respect to the options you present and what they can afford is their responsibility, and theirs alone.

The problem with most clinicians who want to perform more implant procedures—surgical, restorative, or both—has to do with the fact that their ability to perform these procedures far and away exceeds their ability to influence their patients to accept treatment. These clinicians invest mostly in their clinical skill sets through various dental implant continuing education programs only and very little in doctor–patient communications. Yet any clinician I am aware of who has an ability to consistently gain implant case acceptance uses strong visual aids and verbal skills.

If you intend to treat far more patients with dental implants in the coming 12 months, you must refrain from being influenced by thoughts of what your patient can or can't afford and pay far more attention to how you deliver your implant recommendations to the patient.

CHAPTER 2

Patient education seminars

Consumer education seminars have been around for decades, and other industries benefit immensely from leveraging this marketing tool. Real estate investment guru Robert Kiyosaki uses seminars to market his training programs all the time (see Box 2.1). But when I think about how few dental implant providers use this tool as much as experts in other industries, it makes me wonder why.

One of my favorite examples is radio host, *New York Times* best-selling author, and retirement investment advisor Ric Edelman. He has mastered the art of inviting individuals to attend his asset management seminars put on around the country, usually for free or for as little $10–$15. Through his education seminars, Edelman then provides invaluable insight on how to diversify your retirement portfolio through stocks, mutual funds, IRAs, 401Ks, and so on.

He certainly intends to sell books, but the true marketing value in having his firm, Edelman Financial Services, LLC, host these 90-minute seminars is to show its attendees long-term steps they can take to avoid common pitfalls, as well as helpful strategies that may be implemented immediately to set an individual on the right financial path to retirement. The attendee then leaves the seminar feeling more informed about the management of their retirement funds and interested in working closer with Edelman's firm.

Out of a room of 25 seminar attendees, I estimate that if he attracts just two to four new customers who he can serve as clients for years to

Marketing Implant Dentistry: Attract and Influence Patients to Accept Your Dental Implant Treatment Plan, First Edition. Marcus Hines.
© 2016 John Wiley & Sons, Inc. Published 2016 by John Wiley & Sons, Inc.

Box 2.1 Example of investor education seminars used in real estate by Robert Kiyosaki.

Investment education seminars

Real estate investment mogul and author of the *New York Times* bestseller, *Rich Dad Poor Dad*, Robert Kiyosaki, promotes his free seminars on his XM radio talk show. At his seminar, he gives you meaningful information about real estate investing and teaches you how to look for passive-income-earning opportunities. You may leave with a few pearls that can be applied immediately, but much of his goal is to sell his CD recordings, books, or more expensive coaching programs designed to teach the average individual how to buy and sell real estate. If there is true value to be gained, no harm, no foul.

---

come, his firm will profit handsomely and the seminar has served its purpose. The fact that his firm hosts and promotes these seminars to a large listening audience places Edelman Financial Services in what I call the "trusted expert" category. For much of his radio listening audience, this is enough to choose to have Ric Edelman's firm manage their financial assets, whether they attend the seminar or not. His firm claims to have more than 25,000 clients and to manage $14 billion in assets. Edelman is clearly doing something right.

There are thousands of financial advisors who are just as knowledgeable as Edelman, but very few exercise his marketing prowess. The world of implant dentistry is no different. Some clinicians have mastered the consumer/patient education seminar and put up exceptional dental implant numbers as a direct result, but the vast majority do not.

Lasik eye surgery education seminars

More specific to healthcare, when LASIK eye surgery first hit the market in a big way, ophthalmologists were routinely advertising their free patient education seminars on the radio and in newspapers. One of the LASIK surgery companies even hired Tiger Woods to endorse their services. Usually, the eye surgeon giving the seminar would share his credentials, explain to prospective patients the process of LASIK eye surgery, and inform them of the safety, efficacy, and predictability of Lasik eye surgery. The presenter would share supporting statistical data and stroke the prospective patients' emotions by telling attendees that this is their opportunity to rid themselves of those annoying eyeglasses—*for life*. The LASIK surgery candidate would later visit the doctor's office for a consultation that was followed by a $5,000 Lasik eye surgical procedure, which is considerably more expensive than a pair of eyeglasses. Mission accomplished.

Using patient education seminars to attract dental implant patients

Some dental implant cases can be as little as $3,500 for a single tooth or as much as $80,000 for a full-mouth rehabilitation. Many of these patients will arrive in your office ready for treatment, sometimes with little to no one-to-one influential effort on your part. But in most cases, the general public just has a very shallow concept and awareness of dental implants.

Ric Edelman says, "Most Americans have little or no education about money" (Edelman, 2012). Knowing this, he uses his retirement planning seminars to help capitalize on this deficiency. When it comes to implant dentistry, like Ric Edelman, you need to look for every way possible to become a "trusted expert." A part of your mission must be to capitalize on the fact that most people have little or no education about the horrible effects of missing teeth, much less the long-term disadvantages of replacing their missing teeth with more traditional methods, such as partial dentures or full-denture plates. Most people certainly don't understand the exceptional benefits they can gain only by replacing their missing teeth with dental implants.

Patient education seminars can help you capitalize on this deficiency in a big way. Like retirement planning, real estate investments, or before Lasik eye surgery became popular, most people just don't know enough about dental implants to make a sound decision. That said, there are a growing number of people who know enough about the possibility of replacing their missing teeth with dental implants. These individuals are interested to learn more if it means solving the everyday problems they put up with because of their missing teeth.

Out of a group of 15–20 people, you only need two to three individuals to respond positively for your seminars to be worthwhile. For instance, if one seminar attendee receives $6,000 worth of implant-related treatment and another seminar attendee receives $11,000 worth of implant-related treatment, would you consider it worthwhile to routinely host these meetings? The reality is that you will also attract several people who need treatment valued at $25,000 and up. When you promote these seminars in the right way, you will also attract patients in need of dental work that has nothing to do with implant dentistry.

Clinicians like Dr. Frank LaMar of Rochester, NY, has become such an expert at patient education seminars that he now trains other clinicians on performing patient education seminars. The implant numbers such offices produce in implant therapy, year over year, might astonish you. There is no other niche procedure in your practice that will allow you to generate these types of numbers through simply marketing that service to the general public, regardless of your specialty.

If you are a surgical specialist (placing implants only), there is no reason why you too should not offer patient education seminars in your practice. In fact, dental implant seminars may be the only way for you to go directly to the consumer for the purposes of targeting new patients. You can also invite your referring dentists to have their patients attend your seminars as well. Do this and you gain a distinct advantage over your surgical counterparts who refuse to do it or don't know enough about how to conduct these seminars. In Chapter 5, we go deeper into the strategy and rationale for capitalizing on these patient education seminars as a surgical specialist.

Seminar location

If you can hold patient education seminars in your office, you should. Doing so helps establish the relationship in the right way. Prospective patients become familiar with your office in a very nonthreatening way, and you have welcomed these prospective patients into your professional sanctuary, so to speak. And if I were a dentist planning to build out an office, I would make certain that my reception area could comfortably host up to 18–25 people.

Office environment

When the attendees of your patient education seminars show up at your office, it is important that they not feel like they are in a dental office. Think about the makeup of the prototypical person who might attend one of these seminars. A good percentage of these individuals have feared going to the dentist for most of their lives. This has much to do with why they have missing teeth and have chosen not to schedule an appointment directly with an office. You need to be conscious of this.

If your office can facilitate such a meeting, the smell of hard-reline denture material should not permeate the air in your practice, for example. Make sure your office smells fresh. Glade PlugIns are great for treating your air. At minimum, make your office smell very pleasing for these meetings. If you decide to hold these meetings once a month, since the PlugIns are good for about 30 days, your patient education seminars can serve as your barometer for when it is time to replace your refills.

Your office should be clean and well maintained. Your countertops should be clutter-free, your window blinds should be dusted clean, your chairs should be presentable, and the paint and artwork on your walls should appear to be fresh and classy. And if you have a very nice-looking office, these patient education seminars will give you another opportunity to maximize the good money you have invested in your practice by showcasing it to the general public.

Periodontist Dr. Mark Setter is one of the classiest presenters I have had the pleasure of hearing lecture several times. In his lecture titled "Case Acceptance for Contemporary Dentistry," Dr. Setter makes the point that a modern, appealing, and clean office speaks volumes to the patient about the level of service the doctor and his or her staff provide. Having visited hundreds of practices and worked with as many dentists, I must agree with this point.

Although it is not always the case, most times the ambiance of an office will speak to the skill set of the dentist. If your skill set and experience are not adequately represented by the decor of your office, it is most likely costing you in new patient referrals and case acceptance far more than you realize.

If your office is not a good fit for accommodating a patient education seminar, you will be better off holding this meeting at an inexpensive facility nearby that is convenient for people to get to. On the East Coast where I live, we have Wegmans grocery stores, which are so much more than a supermarket. These grocery stores have large sitting areas where you can enjoy freshly cooked, buffet-style meals. Wegmans offers free Wi-Fi service, their facilities are clean, the employees are nice and friendly, and they will usually have a meeting room available that is ideal for the hosting of your dental implant seminars. They can also take care of all of your catering needs as well. Such a location is great because everyone is familiar and enjoys going to Wegmans, and it's convenient because following your presentation, the attendees can plan to pick up a few items from the grocery store if they so choose.

Perhaps you don't have a Wegmans in your area and that's okay. Not everyone can be so lucky! What's important is that you look for a facility with similar characteristics; cost-effective, allows for catering, is easy to get to, and is recognizable. Since many of the prospective patients attending your seminars will be elderly with physical mobility issues, you will want to make sure the facility is handicap friendly.

Refreshments

Be sure to serve nice refreshments including fresh cookies, fresh fruit, juice, and coffee. I also like the idea of serving sandwiches. Sandwiches are a nice touch, and even for the denture wearers who struggle with eating bread, this serves as an envious but tactful and clever reminder that you have a solution to their problems. Again, what's important is that your seminar attendees feel welcomed, almost as if they were visiting a friend's home. Usually, a friend will offer refreshments. So treat these individuals as if they are your dear friends and houseguests.

The presentation

An effective presentation is a must. It doesn't have to be great (at least initially), but it does need to be good. Without a good presentation, nothing I have said or will say in this chapter matters. If you can't influence a reasonable percentage of your attendees to follow your lead and take action, then what's the point of it all? An effective presentation educates the audience first and foremost. An effective presentation will also influence the audience to take action, but does not come off as being too "sales pitchy" or pushy.

The commitment has to be to elevate your audience's dental implant IQ through the presentation in about an hour. If educating your audience remains at the forefront of your mission, your presentation will come across as sincere and the implant patients will follow. That said, don't attempt to make the perfect presentation from day

Box 2.2 The patient education seminar introduction should be more about your staff than you, the dentist.

Example of a patient education seminar introduction

Good evening everyone. My name is Dr. Thomas Smith, and on behalf of my wonderful staff members who I depend on each and every day, I would like to thank you for joining us for this talk on dental implants. This is a procedure that we thoroughly enjoy performing for our patients because, different from a filling or a crown or bridgework or dentures, dental implants have the power to change the quality of an individual's life in an instant. We know this because we have witnessed it happen time and time again with our patients. Later, we'll show you the before-and-after images of a dental implant case we finished for a patient just today, and when we gave her the mirror for the first time, she literally started to cry with tears of joy. ["Lisa, you were able to add Mrs. Jackson's before-and-after images to my presentation, weren't you?" Lisa replies, "Yes, Dr. Smith, they're all there for you." Dr. Smith's response: "You see, I told you how much I count on my staff. (Smiles.) Thank you, Lisa."] And so, I am always honored when our guests show up to listen to me talk about a subject that I enjoy making you aware of. Please make yourselves at home and help yourself to the refreshments throughout this brief meeting. At this point I would like to take a moment to introduce you to our staff:

Lisa is the best when it comes to scheduling patients and making sure that we run on time day-in and day-out. She knows how I can sometimes get caught up in discussions with patients, and if it were not for what Lisa does up front, we would most certainly not run on time in the back. Lisa also coordinates these dental implant open houses for us each month. I don't even have to think about it. If you ever decide to become a patient of our practice, Lisa will be your first point of contact.

Michelle is my dental implant surgical assistant. If I told you all the things she's capable of doing clinically, I wouldn't have time to give my presentation, but Michelle and I have worked together for the past 10 years, and she knows exactly what instruments I need at the precise time that I need them, which makes for a far more efficient dental implant procedure. She takes inventory and orders all of our dental implant supplies, and I never have to wonder if we are prepared for the next dental implant procedure as long as Michelle is around. She knows she's not allowed to leave my side until I retire, which means she's stuck with me for at least another 20 years.

And last but not least is Karen. Karen is my dental implant coordinator who, in fact, works with Lisa to put these meetings together every month. Without Karen, our dental implant operations don't go nearly as smoothly as they do. In fact, Karen is capable of talking to patients about dental implants better than I can. If, for some reason, I couldn't be here tonight, I'm confident the show could go on with Karen as the presenter. She's just a great communicator and has such a vast knowledge about every facet of implant dentistry, which has much to do with why she is so capable of helping patients to understand the different options available to them. Every patient in our practice who is interested in receiving dental implants will eventually have the pleasure of working with Karen.

one. Since there is no substitute for experience, such a task is impossible. The more presentations you give, the more they will evolve. There are steps you can take to reduce your learning curve.

Staff introduction

An effective patient education seminar should start with a warm and friendly introduction of your staff, similar to the outline in Box 2.2. Make it a point to have at least your top three superstars present at every one of these meetings. This might include your implant coordinator, your front desk personnel, and your lead surgical or restorative implant assistant. This is your team, and your audience should have a sneak peek at who they will have the pleasure of dealing with if they should join your practice. This will also help to place your audience at ease and at the same time indirectly promote your practice.

There is no question that patients prefer to be treated by clinically competent and experienced doctors. But your patients also want a dentist who is capable of listening to their concerns, communicates well, and is respectful of their needs and desires, especially when your dental implant procedures are being paid mostly from their hard-earned dollars—not from dental insurance. In other words, patients need to know you care.

A stellar introduction of your staff is important for each of these reasons. Showing your guests that you respect and appreciate your staff a great deal will speak volumes about your personality and the level of respect they can expect as a patient of your practice. If you expect patients to spend $10,000, $25,000, or $60,000 on dental implant services, it helps to show that your staff will play as much of a role as you will in helping each patient travel through this process.

In your introduction, make it a point to spend far more time talking about your staff than you do yourself.

Dentist's introduction

There will be plenty of opportunity to showcase what you are capable of throughout your PowerPoint presentation. The audience knows that you are a dentist; you need to show them you're also human. Therefore, your personal introduction should be geared around your family background (husband/wife, children, etc.), hobbies, extracurricular achievements (marathons, iron man, climbed Mt. Everest, etc.), military service, and such interesting things worth sharing with your audience. Just before you get into your presentation, you will want to share your clinical qualifications. If you are board-certified within your specialty, a fellow or diplomate of AAID, ICOI, and so on, share that information too. If you have placed or restored at least 1000 implants, be sure to share this information as well as to establish your experience.

The introduction you give of yourself should include your qualifications, and it should be the most scripted of each of the introductions, and yet, kept rather brief. Again, your audience will have the body of your presentation to get to know you and what you are capable of.

Who's in your audience and why did they show up?

Now that the friendly environment is set and you have pleasantly introduced yourself and your friendly staff, don't deny your audience the opportunity to introduce themselves if they choose. Ask if there are any individuals in the audience who would like to share what their situations are and why they decided to attend the seminar "this evening." It's also a good idea to ask if there are any medical doctors in the audience. If so, you'll want to make a mental note of these individuals in case they ask questions; you can answer their questions in a way that doesn't make them feel as if you are talking down to them. Let the audience know that you only asked if there are doctors present because much of what you will cover is relative to their overall physical well-being, and no one understands this more than a doctor (physician). Now, your group is set up to be engaged from a much broader prospective.

If you have done a good job to make everyone comfortable with you and the environment, invariably, there will be at least one or two people who eagerly raise their hands and share their situation. I would caution you to be careful not to allow anyone to hog your precious time. After all, the attendees are expecting to be here for an hour to an hour and a half. Therefore, any questions the attendees might pose at this time should be very briefly addressed and politely deferred to the body of the presentation.

The body of your presentation

This is it, the "meat and potatoes" of your presentation. This is what your prospective implant patients came to see you deliver. This is where you showcase your clinical abilities and convince your listening audience that they are in the right place. The body of your presentation is where you will bring everything together.

Topics of discussion
The mood has been well set for your presentation. An effective dental implant education seminar starts with a table of contents or topics of discussion. Before you dig in, tell your audience exactly what you will cover so that they have a map of the road you will take them down, so to speak. Here's an example of what your topics of discussion slide might look like:
- What is a dental implant?
- Why does tooth loss = bone loss?
- Why do we need dental implants to replace missing teeth?
- Dental implants versus fixed or removable bridgework
- Why do dentures become loose over time?
- Full-arch, implant-supported prosthesis (fixed and removable)
- Before-and-after cases
- Common questions and answers

Establish your topics of discussion based on the outline of your presentation, but keep it simple and comprehensive. Once you have established the direction of your presentation, you are ready to get into the body of the meeting.

Include statistical data
Including clinical evidence gathered from research will solidify your message with the audience. Here is where you will want to make your audience aware of some factual evidence, backed by research.

A great one-stop-shop reference guide where you can find all the statistics you'll need for your presentation is in the number one best-selling book on the subject of implant dentistry, *Contemporary Implant Dentistry*, Third Edition, by Dr. Carl Misch (2007). If you don't already have this book, go to www.Amazon.com and order yourself a copy. If you are implant restorative focused, you may be better suited with Dr. Misch's *Dental Implant Prosthetics* (Second Edition 2014) book.

My advice to any dental implant clinician and their staff who is planning to offer these educational seminars is to immediately read chapter 1, "Rationale of dental implants," in either book. Reading this chapter will give you impactful statistical data and references to studies designed to support you in your presentation. This will help you to establish credibility with your audience early on. But be careful not to overload your audience with too much statistical data; to do so would be counterproductive.

What is a dental implant?

It is always best to cover the basics first in any presentation. Explaining what a dental implant is by comparing it to a natural tooth using an image similar to Figure 2.1 is a good place to start. This portion of your

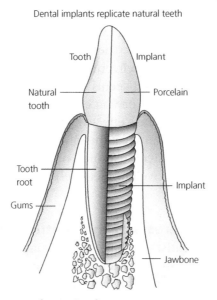

Figure 2.1 A tooth compared to an implant.

Box 2.3 Defining a dental implant should be done early in the presentation.

> ### Scripted definition of a dental implant
>
> Let's start by uncovering exactly what a dental implant is and the main purpose a dental implant serves by first exploring the natural root of a tooth. Virtually every facet of our skeletal system requires stimulation to maintain its shape and form. In other words, if you have ever broken your arm and wore a hard cast for six weeks straight without using that arm at all, you know that the muscle and bone in that arm will shrink and become noticeably smaller than your other arm. This has everything to do with the fact that the broken arm received no stimulation or weight-bearing activity over that six-week period. If you look at the natural tooth [pointing to the left side of the diagram with your laser pointer], it is anchored in the jawbone. Every time we bite and chew our food, the natural tooth root transfers that needed pressure to the surrounding bone and stimulates the jaw. This is how we bring stimulation to our jawbone. Once that tooth root is removed, the underlying jawbone is no longer being stimulated, and therefore, the jawbone begins to shrink at a very rapid rate. Once a tooth is removed, the only way we can regain the stimulating value lost with that removed tooth root is to replace it with an artificial tooth root, called a 'dental implant' [pointing to the implant side on the right].

presentation should be highly scripted as well and should flow something like the example outlined in Box 2.3.

Show me a great salesman and I will show you a person who's mastered the art of delivering a script. The more you deliver the same script, the better you will become at delivering it in a way that influences the listener exceptionally well and seems natural and not scripted at all. Again, you can use this script or you can state it in your own words. What's important is that you are effective at explaining the rationale of a dental implant and that you say it the same way each and every time.

A brief animation that demonstrates bone loss on a partially edentulous arch will serve you well immediately following the delivery of your script.

Speaking to the interests of the denture wearer

I always encourage dentists to share at least one very important statistic about bite forces with their denture patients that resonated with me when I first read chapter 1 in *Contemporary Implant Dentistry*, Third Edition (Misch, 2007). In this chapter, he discusses the scientific rationale for why denture patients experience such a rapid decline in their ability to masticate well.

I encourage you to address some of the larger denture issues in your presentation with passion and empathy, but in a scripted format. Understand what these bite force statistics are for both dentate and edentulous patients so that they roll off of your tongue (see Box 2.4). You may be amazed at the epiphany denture patients in your audience receive once they realize that much of the reason they can't properly chew their food has much to do with the fact that it is nearly impossible, as a denture patient, to adequately retain *bite forces*.

The old adage is true. "When the student is ready, the teacher will appear." Now that you have the denture wearers' (and the would-be denture wearers') attention, you can offer a solution to this horrible debilitation, with passion. At the end of it all, you will passionately offer up a solution to this horrible debilitation.

Sharing these numbers with the right visual imagery can make your presentation strike the perfect chord with denture wearers in their 40s, 50s, and 60s. Statistics are also important for the analytical members of

Box 2.4 Discussing bite forces in a seminar should be highly scripted and accompanied by visual imagery.

Denture patients and bite forces

- An individual with natural teeth will generally exert 150–250 pounds per square inch (psi) bite forces in the first molar region.
- The tissue-borne denture wearer bite forces are only 50 psi in the first molar region.
- The patient who has worn a denture more than 15 years may have a maximum of 5.6 psi bite forces in the first molar region.
- Denture wearers converting to implant-supported teeth may restore their bite forces nearly back to normal (85%) in the first two months of having dental implant-supported teeth.
- It is reasonable to expect the bite forces of the implant patient to ultimately return close to 100% functionality.
- Superior functionality allows the denture patients to chew their food as well as anyone.

Source: *Contemporary Implant Dentistry, 3rd Addition.*

your audience. Most people have never had this information broken down for them in this way as it relates to dentures.

Again, there is a plethora of great statistics you can share with your audience: failed bridgework stats, sinus expansion, absent molar teeth, and so on; just don't overdo it. Three to four impactful statistics can make a big difference in helping you to establish credibility. Keep it as simple as humanly possible. Use phrases like "the back of the mouth" (instead of "posterior"), "bone loss" (instead of "atrophy"), or "chewing power" (instead of "bite forces" or "masticate"). Be conscious of the fact that you're not speaking to a roomful of dental professionals.

Colorful images and animations

If "seeing is believing," then "a picture is worth a thousand words." Call it cliché if you must, but when it comes to patient education seminars, the more images the better. For every meaningful point you make, include an image that says it even better. For example, if you make the point that 25% of the width of bone is lost within the first year following the removal of a tooth, without an image to illustrate this point, your message will fall on deaf ears. But if you can make the same point and demonstrate unmistakable bone loss with an image that even a layperson can appreciate, it will most certainly resonate with your audience, especially the health-conscious females in the group who are actively doing everything possible to avoid the ill effects of osteoporosis.

Don't assume that prospective patients can appreciate what jawbone loss looks like based on your description alone; chances are they will have no idea. So point it out for them in no uncertain terms. Show a side-by-side visual of two mandibles—a healthy mandible with a full set of teeth and the stages of a progressively atrophic edentulous mandible. I promise you this will get their attention. If you ever hope to have a large percentage of your seminar attendees agree to your implant treatment plans, you'll need them to equate tooth loss to bone loss and implants to bone preservation (see Figure 2.2).

Using implant animations adds a visual element

In Oprah Winfrey's interview with Pharrell Williams—the singer, songwriter, and producer of the song "Happy," which ultimately reached #1 on the Billboard Hot 100 List, he tells the story of why, early on, he believed his song was not being played on the radio. Pharrell said months later he cut a video, released the song, and *Boom* everyone loved it! The song hadn't changed, but once the *visual* of the video was released

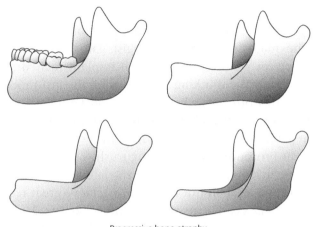

Progressive bone atrophy

Figure 2.2 Progressive bone-loss images help patients understand why dentures are unstable.

to this very catchy tune, it made all the difference—an Oscar and a Grammy award later—and there is no question that a good music video can inspire how you feel about a song.

Appealing to both the *audio* and the *visual* senses can make all the difference in a clinical setting as well. This is the reason I am a huge fan of using animations to educate patients on implant dentistry. A patient education seminar is one place that the right animations can serve its audience well; just don't overdo it with too many animations. For instance, there is no need to show an animation of a ramus graft or sinus lift in this setting. The bone-loss animations are great. Animations showing loss of additional teeth due to failed bridgework are also great. Full-arch, implant-supported prosthetic animations are also great!

Pick and choose your spots for these animations to support your presentation. Two—no more than three—short animations should be all that you need. You never want to rely on too many dental implant animations in your seminars. Only you can truly sell "you"; therefore, keep the animation videos limited.

Before-and-after images

Document, document, document! One of my greatest dental implant-marketing pet peeves is that most clinicians don't take before-and-after images of their dental implant cases. If you consider yourself very good at what you do but you don't take advantage of the priceless gift that every case can offer you, then you really don't get it.

When the mainstream implantologist gains acceptance from a patient to perform an interesting dental implant-related procedure, almost immediately the thinking turns to what the insurance will pay, what the patient's out-of-pocket portion will be, or what materials will bring the most predictable result, and so on. The procedure is performed, the patient is usually pleased, and it's on to the next patient dental implant procedure with nothing to show of the previous case where, in some instances, the surgeon, the lab, and/or the restorative doctor had to "pull a rabbit out the hat" to achieve great results.

When world-class clinicians and presenters like Drs. Michael Pikos, Maurice Salama, Dennis Tarnow, Paulo Malo, Scott Ganz, Hamid Shafie, and others acquire interesting implant cases, I have to believe their thoughts turn to how they will document the journey of their cases from start to finish. On multiple occasions I have heard Dr. Maurice Salama make the point that taking high-resolution images of your cases can help make you a better clinician. Studying your own images gives you the ability to see and improve on flaws that you might have otherwise not noticed.

It requires a different paradigm to envision before-and-after images of a case before ever lifting a scalpel. To think about all the ways you will use such images and compelling patient stories to influence other prospective implant patients or colleagues requires more of a three-dimensional thought process. Whether these exceptional communicators are using their clinical images in a study group setting with a room of 25 doctors or at a lecture in a ballroom filled with 2,500 doctors, everything starts with taking one picture at a time.

You don't have to be world renowned to document your implant cases, but if you're going to conduct patient education seminars, you must begin to build your portfolio one case at a time. You have a congenitally missing maxillary lateral incisor case? At least take pictures before you begin and more pictures when the case is complete. Starting a single-unit, posterior mandible case? Take before-and-after pictures. With every full-arch, immediate-load, or delayed-function case you acquire, plan on taking before-and-after images.

It does take time to document a case, but I promise you, from a marketing perspective, doing so will present you with an invaluable tool for your patient education seminars. When you can show multiple cases that look good and include a compelling patient story, you will be amazed at how easy it becomes to convert many of your audience members into dental implant patients.

Your before-and-after images should include:

• Single-unit, anterior implant case
• Single- or multiunit, posterior implant case
• Full-arch, implant-supported, removable/detachable (Locator®) dentures
• Full-arch, implant-supported, fixed-hybrid case
• 3D treatment planning image

Stay away from using periapicals and panoramic X-rays. In this modern world, HD images can be taken by cell phones, we watch HD televisions, even prenatal ultrasound images are high resolution. A dark, x-ray image that is difficult for the layman to immediately understand will come across as archaic and confusing. If you are an implant surgeon and don't have a CBCT machine, my advice to you would be to use a local mobile unit. If you don't have a local mobile unit available, speak with your colleagues and make arrangements to use a couple of their images in your presentation. All the while realize that this is now considered the standard of care, and ultimately if you are serious about your craft as an implant surgeon, there are few meaningful investments you can make for your implant business that are as worthwhile as a CBCT machine. This is both a clinical and financial asset, not a liability.

Live patient testimonials

It's one thing for an audience to hear you speak about what you can do; it's entirely different to listen to a heartfelt compliment coming from one of your successfully treated dental implant patients. Having a previous implant patient agree to attend the meeting and share the experience with the audience will bring you a profound benefit.

If you have a patient whose overdenture has been stabilized with Locator abutments and you believe she might be willing to offer a testimonial at your seminar, ask her to attend. Once she agrees to do it, and when you're at about the halfway point in your presentation, ask your patient to stand up and share her dental implant experience. This will break the monotony of your presentation and add priceless value instantly. If there is a patient that you performed a full-arch, immediate-occlusal-loading procedure on, ask him if he wouldn't mind sharing

Box 2.5 Nothing beats a great patient testimonial.

Patient testimonials

Hi everyone, my name is Mary Tucker and all of my life I have been very fearful of the dentist. In fact, I lost all of my teeth before the age of 60 and could no longer function with my lower denture. I had gotten to the point that the only time I would tolerate it was when I was in public. But I refused to eat at public restaurants anymore, since I could not chew with my teeth in, which meant I couldn't even go out to eat with my friends. My best friend recommended Dr. Williams after she had received implants. I was still apprehensive, but long story short, I felt as though I had to do something. And I am telling you Dr. Williams's implant surgery was absolutely painless and uneventful. In fact, it happened so fast that I didn't even know we were done until his assistant told me so. I'd say three to four months later, I had my permanent implant teeth, and I'm telling you, these teeth are even better than the teeth I was born with. I can eat anything I want. Just yesterday I had a steak, and today I had corn on the cob. Most of you all look younger than me, but if you should ever need an implant denture, I would strongly recommend Dr. Williams and his staff. I can't say enough about my dental implants.

---

his success story at your seminar. A single-unit, dental implant patient who's willing to share the experience can be just as impactful. Ideally, one or two brief patient testimonials per meeting work best (Box 2.5).

Obviously, you cannot control what your patient will say, nor would you want to. You can control which patients you select to give testimonials. So choose patients who have received the type of implant procedures you are proudest of, choose patients who have received implant procedures you would like to do more of, choose patients who are happiest with their dental implant prostheses and have outgoing personalities, and don't mind expressing their appreciation for what you have done for them.

Nothing beats a live patient testimonial that resonates with members of your audience. Yet for whatever reason, a live patient testimonial may not always be possible. Hence, you will want to make testimonials a part of your PowerPoint presentation. If you haven't already secured testimonials, simply go back to your satisfied implant patients and make the friendly request for a brief testimonial on their experience of receiving dental implant therapy in your practice.

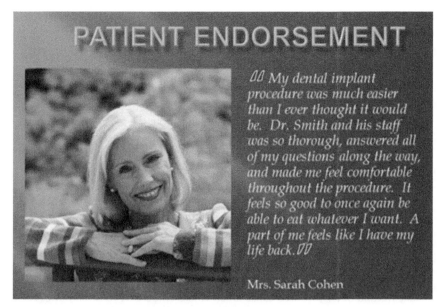

Figure 2.3 Example testimonials in PowerPoint.

Figure 2.3 illustrates an example of what a testimonial slide will look like. A solid three testimonials of this type will serve its purpose well.

Presentation conclusion

I know most dental professionals don't like to think of themselves as salesmen and saleswomen. If this is you, please set this notion aside for just a moment as it will be necessary to use some sales jargon here in order to get my point across in the most effective way.

In the introduction of this book, I stated that in sales, the acronym ABC stands for *Always Be Closing*. You don't have to follow the script as I've outlined it in Box 2.6, but throughout this presentation, you should *always be closing*, particularly at the end of the presentation. Your closing should be very much scripted so that every time you give this seminar, in your conclusion, you are certain to hit on key points that you might otherwise forget to mention.

At this point, you have gone through your presentation as planned, and you could not be more pleased with the way it flowed. The questions asked were intelligent, and you can tell that your responses to

Box 2.6 The patient education seminar closing should tell your audience what the next step in this process is.

Patient education seminar conclusion

On behalf of my staff, I would like to thank each of you for setting aside the time to come out this evening to learn more about replacing missing teeth with dental implants. We are all very passionate about the services we provide here at Pearly Whites Dental Care, and I hope I have shared something of value by explaining the multiple benefits of replacing missing teeth with dental implants, including putting an end to the devastating effects of jawbone loss and regaining the ability to eat virtually any food you desire. I just hope that some of the foods our implant patients choose to eat are healthy foods like raw carrots, nuts, apples, and corn on the cob, if they so choose.

It's very helpful to us if you will take a quick moment to complete a short survey, since we are always looking to improve these seminars. If you are missing one or all of your teeth or you are missing any number of teeth in between, I want to encourage you to stop by the front desk and register with Lisa to take advantage of your free consultation where I'd be glad to sit and discuss your situation and any concerns you might have in more detail, in private. That consultation will be free to you as a thanks for your attendance tonight.

If you feel you are ready for a complete examination and work-up, let Lisa know tonight and she will schedule you for an examination and consultation instead. We'll examine your mouth, take some x-rays, study models, and present you with some options to replace your missing teeth based on what we find during the examination, coupled with your desires. This generally takes about an hour, more or less. And last but not least, we are very proud of our work environment and like to show our guests around, so if you don't mind hanging out with us for just a couple more minutes before you leave, my dental implant coordinator, Karen, would like to give you a brief tour of our facility, and of course, I will be here to answer other questions that might have come up. Again, thank you for coming out, please enjoy more refreshments and I look forward to seeing you in the future.

---

the questions resonated with everyone. The patient testimonials did their part to make many of your guests feel like you should be the person to perform their implant procedures. That said, the success of your meeting should be determined by the number of patients you schedule for a follow-up consultation or examination.

Don't assume that after eating your cookies, drinking your juice and coffee, sniffing your fresh air, and enjoying your presentation, your guests will automatically clamor for an appointment with you. You must tell them what the next step is in this process of replacing their missing teeth. No need to be forceful, but an effective closing will always tell the prospect what the next step should be. You won't monetize these free patient education meetings without a meaningful closing. In this case, you need the prospective patient to understand that the next step in this process is to schedule either a free consultation or an examination and work-up. The better you become at "closing" your presentation in a friendly yet unmistakable way, the better your outcomes will be for each of your meetings.

The postpresentation process

Understanding how your seminar guests feel about your patient education seminar is vital, especially early on. No one will tell you out right that your presentation basically "sucked" and that they got nothing out of it. Chances are most people won't feel that way unless you are really bad, but even if there is one person willing to tell you that there was something in your presentation that he or she just didn't get, most likely someone else missed that same point. Having such feedback allows you to go back and work on that one element so that the next group stands a better chance of understanding your message completely. This is why you must survey your guests.

Survey the attendees
The guests should not feel obligated to identify who they are on the survey. The feedback is more important than anything else, and as with any survey, when people feel like they must identify themselves, they either refuse to complete the survey or they refuse to express how they truly feel. Neither is good. Be sure to survey each attendee before he or she leaves your seminar. Box 2.7 is an example of a survey you can use.

Office tour
Your presentation is complete and your mother would certainly be proud. It's not time to go home quite yet, not before you show your guests around the office. This works best if you have a clear and modern office. Your paint is fresh, your patient rooms are spacious, and your furniture is well maintained. If you have kept up with technology, this is the time to show off your CBCT scanning machine and

Box 2.7 By surveying as many seminar attendees as possible, you position yourself to make improvements in areas you never would have suspected.

Dental implant seminar feedback

Thank you for attending our dental implant seminar. It is our mission to improve our seminar format where possible. Your feedback is invaluable. Please take a moment to answer the following questions:

1 Did you find the information we shared on replacing missing teeth with dental implants helpful?
   ○ Yes   ○ No

2 Did you find the information we shared on bone loss (due to missing teeth) to be informative?
   ○ Yes   ○ No

3 Are you missing teeth, or did you attend this meeting with someone else who is missing teeth?
   ○ Yes   ○ No, attended meeting with someone else

4 How many teeth do you estimate you are missing?
   ○ 1–3   ○ 4–9   ○ 10–14 or more   ○ All upper teeth   ○ All lower teeth

5 Which of the following teeth replacement methods do you currently have? Please check all that apply:
   ○ Fixed bridgework   ○ Removable partial denture
   ○ Full denture plate   ○ None

6 How did you hear about this seminar?
   ○ Radio ad   ○ Newspaper ad   ○ TV commercial
   ○ Friend   ○ I am a patient

7 Has your present dentist talked to you about replacing your missing teeth with dental implants?
   ○ Yes   ○ No   ○ I don't have a dentist

8 Please tell us how you feel about our dental implant seminar overall:
   _____
   _____

---

your in-office crown-milling machine or your digital impression tool. Now is the time to demonstrate why your office is on the cutting edge. Take advantage of the opportunity.

Advertising your patient education seminars

You have carefully planned and crafted your seminar, and now it's time to get it out there. In my opinion, promoting your seminars is the easy part when you consider all that it takes to design and execute one. The reality is that you can't have one without the other.

Postcards to promote seminars to your patient base

There are various ways to use postcards productively in your practice. Promoting your dental implant seminars to your patient base is one of them. You have a captive audience with your patient base, and receiving a postcard in the mail, each and every month, will go a long way towards having your patients understand that you offer dental implant services in your practice.

Virtually every one of your patient's households should receive a postcard promoting your patient education seminar. Even if they cannot attend, the intent is to have your patients know that you are such an expert on this topic that you speak on it each month. You can have the postcards designed and sent out yourself, or you can hire a company to do it all for you. I recommend the latter. When it comes to marketing, the more you outsource, the better your responses will be. Work with a credible company that does this all the time so that your postcards have the best design and they go out automatically every month without you having to think about it.

Some of your patients will attend your seminars, and many more won't. That's okay. Don't take offense or feel as if your efforts are in vain. They're not. Your seminars are primarily about educating, building trust, and attracting new patients. Your patients already trust you, so they may not feel compelled to spend their evening at your office. But this doesn't negate the fact that patients require receiving a constant flow of messages before they will act on their needs. While most of your existing patients won't show up for your presentation, even though they have been receiving and reading the postcards you send out each month, you will recognize how much easier it is to convince your patients of implant treatment when the need presents itself.

How many times have you watched a McDonald's television commercial? Now think about how many times you immediately got off the couch and took your child for a Happy Meal after seeing that McDonald's commercial. Probably never, right? But following your child's

Saturday afternoon soccer game, you make a beeline for McDonald's because he started asking you to take him during breakfast earlier that morning. Understand that this is how marketing and advertising works.

Today, your patient may not need a dental implant, but statistically, rest assured that in the coming months and years she will. And when Mrs. Maxwell is in your office for failed endo or a cracked root or complaints of food impaction around a fixed bridge that probes 9 mm on one of the abutment teeth and you say to her, "It's time to move forward with implants, Mrs. Maxwell," she was already thinking about it before you said it. If you follow the steps outlined in the "Visual aids and verbal skills" chapter, there is a good chance her reply will be "Okay." This is how advertising works.

You know your advertising is effective the moment the consumer recognizes a need and follows through with a purchase. In Mrs. Maxwell's case, it has much to do with the fact that for the last 8 months, she received a irrelevant postcard in the mail from your office inviting her to attend your patient education seminars, which, by the way, she never showed up for. That's when you know your message is resonating with your captive audience. Use postcards to promote implants to your patient base.

Radio advertising

You may be surprised to find out how cost-effective radio advertising can be, depending on the market you serve. There are dentists advertising on the radio all the time in the Washington, D.C., metropolitan area where I live. For years, Dr. Toussaint Crawford (Silver Spring, MD, and Clinton, MD) has advertised on WHUR 96.3 FM, which reaches a large, adult, middle-class, African-American population. Owners of Bethesda Sedation Dentistry, Drs. Deborah Klotz and Robert Schlossberg (Bethesda, MD), target an upper-middle-class audience by advertising on the WMAL 105.9 FM/630 AM radio station.

When you do radio advertising for a service as niche as dental implants, the payoff can be profound. I encourage you to go through an independent advertising agency at least until you believe you know enough to represent yourself. The advertising agent can do all of the groundwork and research for you once you give them the demographics of the patients you are attempting to reach through your radio advertising. You'll also want to work closely with an advertising agent who has a decent amount of experience in representing dentists.

If you are an oral surgeon, you wouldn't advertise third-molar extractions on the radio, nor would you advertise osseous surgery as a periodontist to the general public. How do patients know if their third molars are causing problems or that they have 7 mm pockets without first being examined by their general dentists? They don't. But as discussed in the chapter on "Implant marketing for the surgical specialist," the great thing about advertising dental implant patient education seminars is that all patients are aware of their missing teeth, many are annoyed with their partials, and a large percentage can't eat with their dentures. This is why I love patient education seminars; they're the great equalizer. As a general dentist or specialist, you can advertise these seminars. The invaluable information you provide through your patient seminars will ultimately produce new dental implant patients for you—regardless of your specialty.

Print media

Depending on your marketplace, advertising in the local newspaper may be the way to go for you. The good thing about newspaper advertising is that the age demographic you are looking to attract is most likely still reading the newspaper each day, even in this modern world of the Internet and Twitter. And the amount of people you can draw from a simple newspaper advertisement can be very worthwhile.

Summary

For many years, consumer education seminars have been used successfully across multiple industries, including healthcare, to help bring prospective customers, clients, and patients one step closer to making a purchase. Within the field of dentistry, dental implants might be the best and most fruitful field for such a marketing tool.

With patient education seminars, the goal must always remain to educate the members of the audience. Whether your seminar attendees choose to receive dental implant therapy at your office or not, after leaving your presentation, they should feel like they are much more informed about the prospects of replacing their missing teeth with dental implants.

Strive to put a presentation together that is well scripted, yet flows naturally and does not seem like a sales pitch. About an hour is all the time you need, and if you can offer these meetings once a month within the confines of your office, by all means do so. Use good images that help audience members visually appreciate what you are speaking about, and include before-and-after pictures and two (no more than three) short animations.

Whether you are a surgical specialist or a general dentist choosing to place implants or only restore implants, you can benefit immensely from using patient education seminars in your practice. It is wise to promote your seminars to your patient base. Depending on your market, advertising your patient education seminars to the general public may also serve you very well.

CHAPTER 3

Partnering with physicians for dental implants

Did you ever wonder who the most *trusted* professionals in America are? Teachers? Philanthropists? Spiritual leaders? Dentists are high on the list of trusted professionals as well, but topping this particular list were physicians. According to a 2013 poll conducted by *Reader's Digest* and the research firm The Wagner Group, the professionals most trusted among the general public are medical doctors (Roberts, 2013). And according to the 2010 *Gallup Health and Healthcare Survey*, 70% of Americans are confident in their doctors' advice so much so that they feel no need to seek a second opinion or do additional research on their own (Newport, 2010). This same poll found that 85% of Americans over the age of 65 are confident in their doctors' advice and 67% of those between 50 and 64 have an extremely high regard for their doctors' advice. Simply put, people place extraordinary value on what their doctors tell them to do.

Robin Roberts, cohost of ABC's number one rated morning news show, *Good Morning America*, survived breast cancer, only to be diagnosed with a rare blood disease called myelodysplastic syndrome, or MDS, just 5 years later. This time, her older sister came to her aid with a bone marrow transplant. Now, it appears that she has beaten cancer yet again. In her June 2013 *Reader's Digest* cover story interview, Robin Roberts had this to say of her physician:

"First of all, I think it's very important to develop a relationship with a doctor when you are well. That way, if things do go downhill, you've

---

Marketing Implant Dentistry: Attract and Influence Patients to Accept Your Dental Implant Treatment Plan, First Edition. Marcus Hines.
© 2016 John Wiley & Sons, Inc. Published 2016 by John Wiley & Sons, Inc.

already established "trust." My primary physician has saved my life in so many ways... He's earned my trust."

As much credence as people place on the recommendations of their physicians, it makes you wonder why so few dental professionals ever make a concerted effort to be on the receiving end of a physician's provider recommendation. This is a mistake. If Robin Roberts's physician recommends she see a specific dentist or dental specialist for oral care, how serious do you think she would take that recommendation? Most would agree that she would take her physician's advice to be treated by a specific dental professional, very seriously, to the point of taking action.

A physician's endorsement of you could be priceless

If the mouth is truly the gateway to health, there is no good reason not to target physicians for new patient referrals. Their patients all need your oral care services, and in many instances, the healthcare services physicians provide can be positively impacted by a healthy oral cavity that functions at an optimum level.

I could go on about how periodontal disease has been scientifically linked to everything from low-birth-weight babies to heart disease and diabetes or how denture wearers take higher rates of medication for gastrointestinal disorders. But for the purposes of this book, I will focus here on how you can leverage your clinical skill set and dental implant expertise to educate your medical doctor colleagues on the ill effects of missing teeth and how the patients they treat may also gain health benefits from dental implants.

When you target professionals for dental implant referrals, it is important you shoot for the *quality* in the patient referral, *not the quantity*. Don't concern yourself with large numbers. A very good number for you may be 15 or 20 implant-specific patient referrals, annually, from a collective group of medical providers. Getting to this number won't happen overnight, but it is well worth the effort when you do get there.

Speak in a language the physician understands

Nelson Mandela said, "If you talk to a man in a language he understands, that goes to his head. If you talk to him in his language, that goes to his heart." Be conscious of the fact that each specialty practice is different, and therefore, the provider will respond best to a language they understand based on the type of medical care they provide. Hence, it is your job to tap into the psyche of each of these providers on a one-to-one basis (Figure 3.1).

If, for instance you are particularly knowledgeable on the subject of cancer patients that require being treated with bisphosphonates and what this means for oral surgery, you will benefit to make the local oncologists aware of how you skillfully, tactfully, and cautiously care for your cancer patients who may be receiving oral or IV bisphosphonates or experiencing dry mouth due to the medications.

Why not generate case reports and white papers designed to educate the oncologist from an oral treatment standpoint? "Ten Concerns Every Cancer Patient Should Have About Their Oral Care"

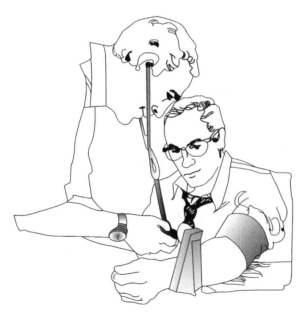

Figure 3.1 Bridging the divide between dentists and physicians is in the patients' best interest.

is an example of a title you might use. If you are an oral surgeon, why would you only think to share these findings with your dental colleagues when so many other healthcare providers can benefit from this information and thus help more patients make the right decision? Share such findings routinely with local physicians and you will become top of mind when a cancer survivor like the aforementioned Robin Roberts requires oral care.

If you're like most dental professionals, you probably look for your new patients in the same old familiar places, each and every month, year after year. A restorative dentist is going to seek out new patients through postcards, examination/cleaning coupons, radio advertising, patient referrals, and so on. The specialist is looking for ways to reach the local restorative dentists, including introducing him or herself to the new dentist in town, running a study group, and inviting restorative dentists to attend in hopes of solidifying relationships, all in the name of maintaining a continuous flow of professional patient referrals. There is nothing at all wrong with any of these methods; in fact, I encourage you to continue such proven efforts if they are bringing you new patients.

But in this increasingly competitive marketplace where patients are better educated and can use this tool called the "Internet" to do their own due diligence on dental implant services before picking up the phone to set an appointment, you had better set yourself up to receive new patients from multiple sources.

Think for a moment what it would be worth to receive a 63-year-old patient referral from an ENT doctor. The ENT doctor recommended his patient see you for an implant consultation because the patient was complaining about an unstable lower denture that's causing sores. Just 1 month later, you receive a 54-year-old, recently divorced female patient referral from the plastic surgeon who has recommended you for a consultation to replace her upper and lower partial dentures with dental implants. Is this possible? Absolutely. It is probable, too, if you will put in the work and plant the seeds necessary to make it happen.

The good thing about reaching out to physicians is that you can do this regardless of being a general practitioner or a specialist. Your goal with such a group should be twofold: (i) You want physicians to recommend your implant services to the patients they treat. And since all people have teeth, including doctors, you also want (ii) these physicians to become patients themselves in your practice when they need to replace their missing teeth with dental implants (more on targeting physicians for their dental implant needs later in this chapter). Now, let's look at how we can attract new patient referrals from medical professionals.

Unconventional methods can lead to extraordinary results

This chapter helps you to begin targeting medical providers in your own town for the purposes of providing dental implants to the patients they care for and, quite frankly, to the physician too. Not every physician will fit this model. And make no mistake, it won't happen overnight, and you will be required to see your marketing efforts through a *different* paradigm. Don't look to your dental counterparts for confirmation, because there is a very good chance that they can't appreciate this strategy if they are not already applying it. You have to be willing to be different in this sense.

The most relevant example I know to offer here is one of myself. I wrote this book because of a desire I felt to serve a larger purpose in implant dentistry than what was possible by representing one implant company through a national position. I knew that if I prematurely shared with colleagues my grandiose ideas about writing a marketing book and starting a podcast, blog, host marketing webinars, and coach implant practices, they would look at me like I was crazy. And who could blame them since there are no examples to draw from? But I avoided negative feedback from individuals not qualified to encourage me which improved my chances of following through. I understood that positioning myself to help so many more dental professionals would require stepping away from the pack and being different.

In her groundbreaking book, *Different: Escaping the Competitive Herd*, Youngme Moon put it this way: "What a breakaway positioning strategy offers is the opportunity to achieve a kind of differentiation that is sustainable over the long term… This, then, is what I mean when I say that breakaway brands succeed in transforming their industries. They leave their imprint by expanding product definitions, by stretching category boundaries, and by forcing competitors to play catch-up for years to come" (Moon, 2010).

Physicians understand the importance of restoring health optimally. What they don't always understand is the importance of replacing missing teeth with dental implants, but this is why they need you to break it down for them. And you can usually relate the ill effects of poor oral health to poor physical health in some way that a physician will appreciate.

Targeting endocrinologists and orthopedic surgeons for patient referrals

Let's first explore targeting orthopedic surgeons. Sharing with an orthopedic surgeon or an endocrinologist images of a severely atrophic mandible (due to lack of stimulation) or images of a patient's CBCT scan that reveals unusually porous bone density will resonate 100% of the time with these doctors. No one understands Wolff's Law, Hounsfield Units and T-scores more than these bone specialists.

In their respective ways, these physicians specialize in treating the musculoskeletal system. And because you, too, deal with bone and medical devices, and must at least be aware of a dental implant candidate's use of bisphosphonates, you share this unique commonality with orthopedic surgeons and endocrinologists. So, let's look deeper into how you can use this potential rapport builder for the good of your patients, the physicians' patients, and your practice.

With all that an orthopedic surgeon understands about bone, you still may need to make him or her conscious of the fact that the lower one-third of the face requires either the natural tooth root or an artificial root to transfer stimulation from the crown of a tooth to the jawbone, if both form and function of the jaw is to be maintained. The best way I know to do this is with very good dental implant animated software designed to illustrate exactly what happens to the jawbone of denture wearers over time. You need to give the physician a sense of what patients witness when they go through your implant consultation, which is all the more reason to invite these practitioners to your office for a tour.

When establishing these relationships, your patients' health must remain at the forefront of your motivation. Your mission should be to expand your healthcare resource pool even more so than it is to expand your new patient referral base. This requires that you understand what medical care your targeted physicians offer their patients. The more you can separate yourself from the typical oral healthcare provider by becoming more of a healthcare resource for your patients and physician colleagues, the more professional patient referrals you will receive.

For instance, let's consider endocrinologists. According to the National Osteoporosis Foundation, nearly 9 million US adults suffer from osteoporosis, and 48 million adults suffer from low bone density. Worldwide, 200 million are afflicted with osteoporosis. Each year, there are 2 million broken bones and $19 billion in related costs because of osteoporosis. Endocrinologists and orthopedic surgeons are faced with an enormous epidemic.

This is a major healthcare issue, but an issue that, quite possibly, you can help certain patients in your practice prevent by paying attention to the bone density through the CBCT scans you take and the tactile feel of unusually low bone density you experience when drilling your osteotomies in, say, the lower anterior region. This may be the best early sign of low bone density your young and otherwise healthy 24-year-old patient will offer to any clinician before actually breaking a bone. Her best opportunity to get checked by an endocrinologist might be from your recommendation.

The physician's diagnosis of the patient you referred could be as severe as osteoporosis or a less harsh diagnosis, which can lead to recommendations as simple as dietary changes and more low-impact exercises including dialing back the black-diamond skiing activities a bit, as an example. Point is, because of your attentiveness and call to action, your patient might be able to do something about this problem before it worsens or, at minimum, take certain physical activity precautions. Of course, it could turn out that there is no problem at all. Nonetheless, the information you are privy to as an implant surgeon can potentially make a huge impact on your patients' overall health.

So, what does this all have to do with marketing? I've said it before and I'll say it again: Patient care must always be first and foremost. Then, it becomes a process of reciprocity. If you want to receive professional referrals, you too, must refer. And if you will expand your network to include orthopedic and endocrinologists surgeons for the benefit of your patients, you stand to gain a tremendous marketing advantage over your dental professional colleagues whose patient referral network is limited almost exclusively to other dental

Box 3.1 Introductory letter to local orthopedic surgeon.

Example letter to orthopedic surgeon

Dear Dr. Orthopedic Surgeon [personalize],

I am a local dentist with a practice emphasizing implant dentistry. As the demographics of my patient base continue to age, I recognize a growing prospect in some patients that might make them a candidate for joint surgery such as knee and hip replacements.

I would like an opportunity to speak with you in the near future to gain a better understanding of the signs and symptoms to look for that might warrant referring a patient to an orthopedic surgeon for a consultation. Eventually, I would also like to share with you some approaches we take to regenerate atrophied areas of the jawbone in order to replace missing teeth with medical devices known as dental implants.

If it works for your schedule, I would like an opportunity to meet with you. I will contact your office in the next few days to introduce myself. Thank you for your consideration, and again, I hope to get together soon.

Sincerely,
Dr. Implant Dentist

---

professionals and patients. This is why it is vital that you get to know these doctors first. You can begin by mailing a letter similar to Box 3.1 to virtually every orthopedic surgeon in your area. If mailing to an endocrinologist, your letter will be slanted toward osteoporosis.

Such a letter is effective when it outlines your mission, is brief, and straight to the point. Tell the doctor what you do, and more importantly, show respect for what they do. Don't expect this letter to garner an immediate and enthusiastic response from every orthopedic surgeon you send it to. But it is a very good way to break the ice and begin cultivating a relationship.

Targeting the gastroenterologist doctors

Since the mouth is where the physical digestive process begins, shouldn't oral healthcare providers and gastroenterologists have a much closer working relationship?

My 64-year-old brother-in-law, Sloan, wore an upper and lower complete denture for close to 25 years. At a family gathering, I noticed that Sloan would chew his food, and before swallowing, he would immediately take a gulp of his beverage in an effort to make the process of swallowing more tolerable. I should add that for years Sloan has suffered from heartburn and acid reflux.

One year after receiving 11 implants, and an upper and lower implant-supported, fixed-hybrid prosthesis, his instances of heartburn had noticeably been reduced, and his dependence on medication for acid reflux had also decreased. Coincidental? Based on the literature, one would have to presume not. I imagine his bite forces have been completely restored to his predenture wearing years because he says he can't remember when he has chewed his food so well and that he no longer needs water to assist him with swallowing. The irony is that the strong recommendation for dental implants came from me, a non-clinician, not his gastroenterologist.

Gastroenterologists may specialize in treating symptoms associated with the digestive track including heartburn, indigestion, difficulty swallowing, and so on, but are most of these physicians consciously aware of the fact that the average new denture wearer retains only about 20–33% (or 50 psi) of a natural ability to chew and grind their food before swallowing? Are they consciously aware that 17% of denture wearers say they chew better without their prosthesis (Misch, 2007)? It's certainly well documented in the literature, but I have to believe that they simply don't understand enough about the digestive benefits that many of their patients can gain from an implant-supported prosthesis. Why didn't Sloan's gastroenterologist give him a prescription for Prilosec®, an implant brochure, and a referral form that included a complimentary consultation with the dental implant specialist who rents office space in the same medical park as he, the gastroenterologist, does?

We cannot expect gastroenterologists to refer their patients to an oral healthcare provider for dental implants if we aren't willing to help them establish and maintain a certain level of awareness. If you truly desire to use your skill set to help more people improve their health and quality of life, dramatically, make an effort to be top of mind to the gastroenterologists in your town when it comes to their denture-wearing patients, and you can do it with little to no competition. To do so will require that you first educate them on the facts about tissue-borne, denture-wearing patients starting with the fact that they take significantly more medication than individuals with superior masticatory abilities.

Box 3.2 Introductory letter to local gastroenterologist.

Example letter to gastroenterologist

Dear Dr. [personalize],

I am a local dentist with a practice emphasizing implant dentistry. Over the years, I have recognized that my denture patients have noticeably higher instances of gastrointestinal disorders compared to patients with natural teeth. The literature demonstrates that denture wearers take significantly more medication (17% more) compared to people with natural teeth or normal chewing abilities.

I am reaching out to you in an effort to become more knowledgeable about this disorder, so that I can be of better service to my patients. I also believe that my dental implant practice might serve as part of the prescribed solution to many patients who happen to wear dentures. We have more than a 95% success rate in helping denture patients restore their chewing abilities to normal, which can have an enormous effect on their ability to grind, swallow, and digest their food more efficiently.

If it works for your schedule, I would like an opportunity to meet with you. I will contact your office in the next few days to introduce myself. Thank you for your consideration, and again, I hope to get together soon.

Sincerely,
Dr. Implant Dentist

Consider sending the letter in Box 3.2 to this group, on your letterhead. A variation of this letter should be sent to virtually every gastroenterologist in your marketplace to open doors and to begin establishing relationships. If you are only planning to use this tool once or twice to reach out to these professionals, don't bother. Such a limited effort won't be worth your time or money because you most likely won't receive much of a reaction.

Educate this group on how crippling an ill-fitting denture can be to a patient's ability to adequately begin the digestive process. Document your full-arch implant cases well. Share with these physicians your full-arch, dental implant-supported cases, including fixed and removable, and their success stories. Become a resource and team member in the eyes of the gastroenterologist when it comes to helping rehabilitate their denture-wearing patients' lost ability to chew and swallow their food well. Do this and you open yourself up for an untapped, yet powerful implant referral source.

Targeting otolaryngologists (aka ENT doctors)

Physicians like otolaryngologists (ENT) also offer a promising opportunity to elicit patient referrals, but in a different way. Since these doctors specialize in treating the head, neck, and throat and routinely treat the sinus region, they can be a great clinical resource to leverage.

Perhaps this group of physicians asks their patients to "open wide" nearly as often as you do. They're looking at tonsils, reviewing images of sinuses, surveying the palate, addressing sleep apnea, caring for TMJ, and indirectly taking notice of loose-fitting dentures every day in their practices. The more comprehensive ENT doctors will be encouraged when you speak their language and show a sincere desire to build a reciprocal relationship.

Periodontist and author of four soft tissue- and dental implant-related textbooks, Dr. Lee Silverstein and his coauthor and partner Dr. Peter Shatz, out of Atlanta, GA, encourage dentists in their lectures to work closely with ENT and other physicians in the best interest of the patient.

Dr. Randolph Resnik, a prosthodontist with a private practice in Pittsburg, PA, and a well-respected authority in CBCT-based diagnosis and treatment plan training, is as big of an advocate on sharing patient referrals with ENT doctors as I have seen. In a case report he penned for the journal *Implant Practice*, July/August 2014, titled CBCT – Not So Incidental Findings, Dr. Resnik said, "By having the patient treated and cleared for future procedures in the maxillary sinus with an ENT, the implant dentist has the ability to form a relationship with an ENT physician that will be crucial if postoperative complications develop" (Resnik, 2014). It is easy to understand the reciprocal benefits associated with routinely referring patients to an ENT doctor for sinus-related matters, but what is most evident is that the patient's best interest is at heart, first and foremost. Then patient referrals can follow.

Most dentists don't keep in touch with denture patients very well, long term. Consequently, patients with old, ill-fitting dentures tend to show little commitment to their current dentists and therefore have no problem with changing dentists at a moment's notice—bad for a patient's current dentist, but works like a charm for you, if you create a funnel system for attracting such patients. Like Dr. Resnik, one way to do this is to establish relationships with ENT doctors. Look for opportunities to benefit your patients in need by referring them to an

ENT, and educate the ENT on how you can benefit their patients that happen to wear a tissue-borne denture. They see these cases all the time, and when the ENT recommends their denture-wearing patients see you for an implant consultation, these patients will follow suit.

Consider sending a variation of the sample letter in Box 3.3 to most ENT doctors in your surrounding market, followed by setting up meetings with these doctors. Develop an understanding for each ENT's treatment philosophy. Share your approaches to treating patients with dental implants and how the sinus must sometimes be augmented for an optimal result. Communicate your intentions for referring out your patients with sinus concerns. Over time, continue to educate the ENT doctor on the by-products of missing teeth and ill-fitting dentures due to bone atrophy. Not every ENT doctor will appreciate your vision of sharing patient referrals, and that's okay. You are in pursuit of the one, two, or three that will.

Once relationships are established, supply the ENT doctors with dental implant patient educational brochures with your contact information preprinted on the brochures. Describe the type of patient an ENT doctor should refer for an implant consult, assure he or she that you will evaluate their patients' dentures, recommend a treatment

Box 3.3 Introductory letter to local otolaryngologist.

Example letter to ENT doctors

Dear Dr. ENT [personalize],

I am a local dentist with an emphasis in caring for patients with dental implants. In treating patients with maxillary dental implants, the condition of the sinus cavity cannot be ignored and oftentimes must be augmented. Many of my prospective dental implant patients are afflicted with sinus infections, and I believe, in multiple cases, such patients would benefit from the aid of an otolaryngologist.

I would like an opportunity to meet with you and to review some of the sinus conditions I find my patients in and would like your opinion on which conditions are better off being referred to an otolaryngologist for treatment.

If it works for your schedule, I would like an opportunity to meet with you. I will contact your office in the next few days to introduce myself. Thank you for your consideration, and again, I hope to get together soon.

Sincerely,
Dr. Implant Doctor

resolution, and communicate your recommendations back to the referring ENT. And remember, this is a marathon, not a sprint.

Targeting plastic surgeons for patient referrals

Plastic surgeons are caring for patients that want to look and feel better about themselves and want facelifts, nose jobs, breast implants, Brazilian Butt Lifts®, and so on. Restored self-confidence, in part, is the modus operandi of the cosmetic patient that plastic surgeons treat every single day of the week. Having a very good plastic surgeon as a resource will prove profitable over time. I would encourage you to send virtually every plastic surgeon in your town a letter similar to the example in Box 3.4.

Consider the influence a plastic surgeon has over the 52-year-old male patient with a successful career in physical training and public speaking. A person of this career path can easily find himself in a midlife crisis, desiring to have a face-lift. Or think about the 56-year-old mother of three and successful business owner who is increasingly conscious

Box 3.4 Introductory letter to local plastic surgeons.

Example letter to plastic surgeons

Dear Dr. [personalize],

I am a local dentist with a practice emphasizing implant dentistry. As my patient population continues to age, I recognize an increasing desire to retain a youthful appearance, among my aging patients. Consequently, as their trusted oral care provider, I realize the benefit it would mean to many of my patients if I were to maintain a close working relationship with an experienced plastic surgeon. For this reason, I would like to meet with you soon.

At some point, I would also like to share examples of how we are able to help esthetically driven patients, who happen to be missing teeth, improve the lower one-third of their facial profile, reestablish lip support, and replace missing teeth, all with the aid of implant dentistry.

If it works for your schedule, I would like an opportunity to meet with you. I will contact your office in the next few days to introduce myself. Thank you for your consideration, and again, I hope to get together soon.

Sincerely,
Dr. Implant Dentist

of more facial wrinkles and is now adamant about going under the knife.

Statistically speaking, chances are both 50-something patients are missing multiple teeth and may even be wearing a partial denture or a complete denture. In addition to opting for facial plastic surgery, such patients can easily be influenced by their plastic surgeon to also consider replacing their missing teeth with dental implants in an effort to stop the jawbone loss that can influence premature facial aging.

Targeting obstetrician and gynecologists (OB/GYN)

With OB/GYN practitioners, your mission has more to do with establishing a relationship and much less about directly seeking implant patient referrals. Establish a meaningful relationship based around your exceptional attentiveness to the oral care services of expecting mothers, and the implant patients will follow, mostly as an indirect result.

My sister-in-law, Dr. Brenda Hines, a board certified obstetrician and gynecologist, says many of her gynecological patients routinely happen to be looking for a "good dentist." Dr. Hines says, "Periodically my patients will ask me to recommend a dentist for various reasons. But in my 20 years of private practice, I haven't been formally solicited by a dentist or a dental specialist for the purposes of patient referrals."

In a 2013 report produced by The American College of Obstetricians and Gynecologists titled Oral Healthcare During Pregnancy and Through the Lifespan, the authors state: "Although most obstetricians acknowledged a need for oral health care during pregnancy, 80% did not use oral health screening questions in their prenatal visits, and 94% did not routinely refer all patients to a dentist."

The reality is that the same aforementioned 94% of OB/GYNs that do not routinely refer patients to a dentist, would also include not referring the hypothetical pregnant patient who is newly relocated, has gums that are severely inflamed, suffers from lower levels of calcium, and is in jeopardy of losing at least one tooth during her pregnancy if immediate action isn't taken.

Box 3.5 Example of an introductory letter to an OB/GYN.

Example letter to OB/GYN

Dear Dr. OB/GYN [personalize],

I am a local dentist with an emphasis in implant dentistry. As you may know, periodontal disease is the number one reason patients lose their teeth. The linkage of periodontal disease to low birth weight in infants is also well documented in the literature.

Many of our expecting dental patients suffer from inflamed gums and increased caries, and others lose teeth unnecessarily. In an effort to improve my service to this segment of my patient base during pregnancy, I would like an opportunity to meet with you. I am also asked by my patients to recommend an obstetrician for various reasons from time to time and would like to understand your practice philosophy.

If it works for your schedule, I would like an opportunity to meet with you in the near future. I will contact your office in the next few days to introduce myself. Thank you for your consideration, and again, I hope to get together soon.

Sincerely,
Dr. Implant Dentist

Is your relationship with this patient's OB/GYN strong enough that you are top of mind for a patient referral? Does this patient's OB/GYN understand that you will see any of her patients referred for periodontal concerns, on the same day? And are you willing to initiate a lunch meeting with the OB/GYN to review X-rays and images, discuss the urgency of care and health history, and gain consensus on local X-ray and anesthesia protocols based on this patient's specific needs? How significant of a healthcare provider do you become in the eyes of the obstetrician for future patient referrals if you are willing to go to this extent?

The periodontist, in particular, may begin cultivating a relationship with obstetricians by consistently keeping these physicians conscious of the well-documented, ill effects periodontal disease is known to have on pregnant women and their fetuses. And when you receive these types of physician referrals, following (or during) your periodontal treatment of the patient, as a specialist you suddenly have the ability to recommend this patient to a restorative dentist from within your network.

These patients trust their OB/GYNs and thoroughly respect their professional recommendations, as they should. And most any OB/ GYN can appreciate the improved health of the mother, her fetus, and eventually the newborn child when good periodontal health is achieved.

Your goal is to educate the OB/GYN on your practice philosophy when it comes to caring for expecting mothers. You may be surprised at how much respect a simple letter, like the example in Box 3.5, can garner from the OB/GYN professional community. TV personality and cardiothoracic surgeon, Dr. Mehmet Oz, MD, routinely talks about multiple systemic issues tied to periodontal disease. And since many of these patients are missing at least one tooth, you set yourself up to be their dental implant provider as well, following the birth of their child.

Other healthcare providers to target

This is only the tip of the iceberg in terms of the types of healthcare providers you'll want to establish a reciprocal relationship with for the purposes of ultimately receiving dental implant patient referrals. Other providers that should also be on your radar include dermatologists, chiropractors, naturopaths, ophthalmologists, podiatrists, urologists, hand doctors, and nutritionists.

Think about what nutritionists gets paid to do. Essentially, a major part of their skill set is geared around educating people on what foods to eat in order to lead healthy lives. These respected professionals encourage their clients to eat certain meats and nuts for protein and raw fruits and vegetables for valuable vitamins and fiber content. Physicians like endocrinologists, oncologists, and cardiologists refer a great deal of their patients to nutritionists.

A 62-year-old, obese patient (and denture wearer) is afflicted with type 2 diabetes, hypertension, and clogged arteries, for example. After receiving a successful triple bypass, open heart surgery, his cardiologist then recommends that the patient consider gastric bypass surgery and referrers him to an experienced plastic surgeon specializing in this procedure for a consultation. The cardiologist also recommends that his patient adopt a diet that includes adequate amounts of raw fruits, vegetables, and nuts. Happens all the time. But what if the patient's ill-fitting lower denture won't allow him to eat the recommended food types or even sufficiently chew the foods he enjoys, like poultry and steak? Is it top of mind for this cardiologist to also refer his patient for a dental implant consultation? Most likely not.

All types of physicians are routinely faced with opportunities to better serve their patients by referring them to an oral healthcare provider. Being on the receiving end of physician patient referrals will require you to put in the effort to educate your local medical community on the profound effects implant dentistry can play in a patient's overall health. Do this properly, and in the eyes of the local physician, you become the expert go-to person for this and other treatment modalities.

Keep your expectations realistic

Will any one OB/GYN, dermatologist, or cardiologist ever refer you 20 or 30 patients per year? Assuming you're married to one—maybe. Otherwise, most likely not, so don't set yourself up to expect it. Obviously, physicians are not in the business of managing their patients' oral health, so keep your expectations low about the number of patient referrals you might receive from any given physician or you might become disappointed, and that disappointment might lead you to make an ill-advised decision to cease all efforts at targeting this group.

But is it possible to receive 10–15 or more *quality* dental implant patient referrals each year from a group of physicians in your area? Absolutely! And it is well within reason for five or six of these patients to be worth $20,000, $30,000, $50,000, or more in dental implant treatment needs. The other patients might be worth closer to $10,000 or $12,000 or more in dental implant therapy, not to mention all the other oral care needs many of these patients will have.

The fact that a patient is being referred by a physician for oral care means that it's probably not for a single posterior molar tooth. Chances are the patient has other underlying health issues that have caused the physician to view their oral condition as a significant hindrance to the process of achieving long-term health. Therefore, it is not the lower volume of patient referrals that should concern you. The quality of the patient referral is what you must pay attention to.

Physicians need dental implants too

As much as I am an advocate for partnering with physicians in the best interest of the patient, I am just as much of an advocate of targeting physicians for their personal dental implant needs, too. It doesn't matter how you slice it—70% of all Americans are missing at least one tooth, including physicians.

These are individuals that understand how the body works and won't require as much of an explanation to appreciate just how profound the process of replacing missing teeth with dental implants really is. Additionally, they make good money and, in most instances, should be able to afford your treatment plans.

According to Salary.com, orthopedic surgeons' earnings are among the highest of all physicians, as seen in Table 3.1. The question isn't if these high six-figure salary earners can afford your services—because they can. The better question is whether or not you are capable of influencing them to receive the treatment they need, at your practice.

Couple this with the fact that nearly one-third of all adults in the United States between the ages of 55 and 64 suffer from mandibular free-end edentulism, why wouldn't you target this group of health-care providers for dental implant therapy? They have mandibular free-end edentulous sites, too. They will respect you as a fellow clinician. They can appreciate a well-thought-out treatment plan. And they are easy to find in any town. Call up any list broker, and they'll tabulate a list of physicians, sell it to you, and have it in your e-mail box faster than you can take a lunch break.

Even if the cardiologist has a dentist that he or she happens to be pleased with, strategically targeting these healthcare providers in

Table 3.1 Some specialized physicians salaries.

Median annual salaries	
Orthopedic surgeon	$434,163
Plastic surgeon	$346,408
Gastroenterologist	$342,413
Urologist	$338,976
Otolaryngologist (ENT)	$331,101

Salary.com. Last accessed March 2015.

the right way might still lead a certain percentage to come to your office for their dental implants if they believe you are particularly skilled in that area. And having the medical provider as a patient in your practice increases the chances of that provider recommending you to their patients.

Comarketing efforts

Consider doing some comarketing with other healthcare providers. For example, you might invite your trusted cardiologist and registered nutritionist to head up a heart-healthy session hosted by you at your office. Send a letter of invitation to every 45-year-old and older patient in your practice to join you in this session. Promote the session on your website and through your social media outlets. Send out postcards to the surrounding adult population with the details, and ask them to contact your office to RSVP for this free event. The RSVP will give you an idea of what your turnout will be.

Have the cardiologist and his nurse screen attendants for high blood pressure, listen to their concerns, check their heart rates, make general recommendations, and provide take-home supportive materials that should include contact information for the cardiologist's private practice. The registered nutritionist should be on hand to offer dietary advice on recommended foods for individuals with heart-related concerns.

Set it up so that this is an annual event in your office. And you don't have to limit the event to just one area of medical treatment. Select a different type of healthcare provider and hold such an event in your office twice a year. I don't really recommend more than two, because if you promote each event properly, it will take time and effort to pull it off. Besides, each month you have your patient education seminars to plan for, too (see Chapter 2). The key is to target those individuals with the greatest potential need for dental implants. The more prospective implant patients walking through your office, the better.

Whatever you do, don't lose sight of the end goal. When you hold these events, do all you can to promote the healthcare provider who has agreed to team up with you—not your practice. Your goal should be to attract as many patients as possible for that medical provider for two reasons: (i) Patient health must be at the heart of every event, and (ii) the more your event assists the physician in his effort to attract new patients, the more anxious the physician will be to reciprocate in a similar fashion.

In the earlier example, your strategy must be to have your partnering cardiologist send out a letter to his patient base inviting them to attend a similar event that would be held at *the cardiologist's* office, but this time on your behalf. For instance, you might offer to provide a free denture or dental implant, oral health screening of sorts. Most patients hold their cardiologists in very high esteem. For this reason, such an event will certainly serve you well in your effort to attract prospective dental implant patients.

Summary

Oftentimes, oral healthcare professionals forget the fact that the mouth is the gateway to good health and that the mouth, in so many ways, is connected to most every facet of our overall physical well-being. And in many instances, the literature validates the fact that a poor state of oral health can be a significant contributor to various, poor physical conditions.

Dental professionals who are willing to take a systematic approach toward partnering with medical providers for the purposes of both referring out, and receiving patient referrals, will position themselves to tap into a whole new resource of quality, new patients who are ideal candidates for receiving multiple dental implants. There are countless ways a dental professional can partner with a physician to attract more patients who are in need of dental implants. With a little creativity and consistency, this untapped market can generate a consistent stream of professionally referred dental implant patients.

CHAPTER 4

Marketing full-arch implant dentistry in your practice

One of the most difficult things for me to wrap my mind around is how challenging it is for so many dentists to see a traditional *tissue-borne denture* as being little more than a short-term solution, much less obsolete. Maybe the fact that I'm not a dentist has something to do with it, except that many of my dentist clients and dentist friends also struggle with the fact that the denture is still far and away the number one solution offered to edentulous patients by their colleagues.

Back in the late 1700s when pioneering dentist Dr. John Greenwood designed President George Washington's first set of dentures, this was cutting-edge know-how. The teeth may have looked as though they were made from wood, and the esthetics left much to be desired, but it was certainly better than the alternative of having no teeth at all.

Even the most modern-day, superior denture design using the principles taught by the renowned Dr. Jack Turbyfill still has its limitations. After all, a denture isn't anchored in bone as natural teeth or dental implants are. Consequently, jawbone atrophy is still just as predictable for edentulous patients as it was back in the 18th century.

What other industry can you think of that embraces such an old concept over a modern, innovative alternative as much as dentistry continues to embrace the denture, in spite of its inferiority to the more

Marketing Implant Dentistry: Attract and Influence Patients to Accept Your Dental Implant Treatment Plan, First Edition. Marcus Hines.
© 2016 John Wiley & Sons, Inc. Published 2016 by John Wiley & Sons, Inc.

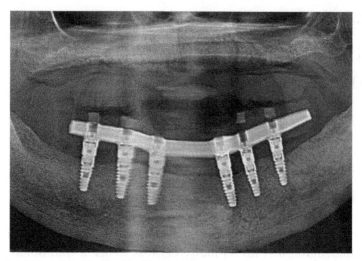

Figure 4.1 Before/after lower fixed hybrid and upper denture. Dr. Thuan-Anh Nguyen, General Dentist (Wheaton, MD), and Dr. Charles Chen, Periodontist (Olney, MD). Reproduced with permission of Dr. Nguyen.

advanced dental implant-supported prosthesis such as in Figure 4.1? You would be hard-pressed to find one.

Consider the old automobile bumper designs. When I was a child, my father had a 1976 Buick Electra with big and bulky chrome bumpers that protruded out from the car and served little more purpose than to minimize front and back end damage. Today, bumpers aren't designed to protect the car as much as they are programmed to save our lives. Front bumpers are now equipped with sensors that require less than a 10th of a second to deploy air bags and cushion the driver and passengers' heads from the trauma of the steering wheel, dashboard, and side impact. Because of this engineering marvel, more than 28,000 lives have been saved over the course of its first 30 years (NHTSA, 2014). Rear bumpers house sensors designed to alert the driver when they have backed too close to an object, parked car, or worse, a small child. Who wouldn't insist on such advancements in an automobile today?

It doesn't matter the industry. Whether it is eliminating lead from paint and gasoline, the use of smartphones, or making medical advancements that helps to preserve the quality of life, thank goodness that in many ways we are no longer forced to resort to old and limiting solutions.

Even in dentistry, most practices have gone from the time-consuming manual X-rays to having a computerized digital PA image, instantly. Today, you can prep a tooth and deliver the final crown on the same day. When planning for implant surgery, the limiting two-dimensional panoramic image that often left you playing guessing games has taken a backseat to the superior three-dimensional treatment planning capabilities of a CBCT scan.

Name a meaningful product that has been around for less than half as long as the denture, including medical devices, and I will show you multiple examples of products that have been dramatically improved or deemed obsolete. When will the dental profession at large classify the denture obsolete as a long-term solution to edentulism?

Tissue-borne dentures: The short-term solution

Many dentists and maybe even laboratory technicians reading this chapter may criticize me for lumping tissue-borne dentures with "chromed auto bumpers" and "leaded paint," but I have a very good excuse for doing so. I never had the benefit of attending dental school, so I don't understand the true essence and worth of a good quality denture.

Obviously, there is still a place in dentistry for a well-made, tissue-borne denture. I believe this in spite of the numerous, well-documented disadvantages of wearing one. Some of these disadvantages are listed in Box 4.1. As a rule, I just don't believe the denture should be presented to the patient as if it were a long-term solution to edentulism, regardless of their financial wherewithal.

It is true that not every patient faced with edentulism can afford an implant-supported prosthesis, right here and now. And such patients should be presented with the option of having a tissue-borne denture— with one caveat. I believe an attempt should be made to help every edentulous patient to thoroughly understand the masticatory disadvantages of wearing a traditional tissue-borne denture, long term. What's wrong with telling your patient what you already know? Your patient needs to know that if not properly treated, edentulism is a very bad healthcare problem that worsens with time.

Box 4.1 Statistical data at key points in a doctor–patient conversation can be impactful.

Influential facts about denture wearers

- The average first-molar-region bite forces in dentate patient is 150–250 psi
- The average maximum bite forces in the edentulous patient is less than 50 psi
- The maximum bite forces in denture patients of more than 15 years is 5.6 psi
- Seventeen percent claim to eat more efficiently without dentures
- Twenty-nine percent are able to eat only soft or mashed food
- A removable denture accelerates bone loss
- Forty percent of denture wearers have worn an ill-fitting denture for more than 10 years

Source: *Contemporary Implant Dentistry, 3rd addition* (Misch, 2007)

It is in the patient's best interest to have the long-term, negative effects of wearing a denture spelled out both verbally and in the doctor's consent form. For example, "A denture might contribute to or accelerate jawbone loss over time" or "When worn long term, a traditional tissue-borne denture might lead to substantial jawbone loss and limit the ability to adequately chew food."

Patients who find it difficult to pay for dental implants all at once should be encouraged to take a staged approach. With this in mind, your denture disclaimer might also encourage dental implants by saying something like: "We encourage most denture patients to transition from a traditional 'tissue-borne denture' to an 'implant-supported denture'" or "A 'dental implant-supported denture' may help prevent significant jawbone loss and maintain the ability to properly chew food long term."

As much as I am not a dentist, neither am I a lawyer. Therefore, seeking legal advice should always be a top priority anytime you construct a disclaimer or consent form. These are only suggestions for the tone of your messages to the patient. That said, the more you project the denture as a *short-term* solution, the more you will watch your full-arch, dental implant-supported prosthetic numbers increase. Many patients will immediately opt for immediate load, while other patients will stage their process of receiving implants over the course of 2, 5, or even 8 years. Either way, the patient is far better off long term.

In my experience, patients can afford a full-arch, implant-supported prosthesis far more often than the typical dentist believes. The bigger problem has more to do with the fact that most dental professionals don't understand how to encourage full-arch, dental implant-supported prostheses in their practices nor do they understand how to talk to these patients about supporting their full-arch denture with dental implants in a commonsense way the patient can appreciate from an intellectual prospective. It's about empathy and being compelling in your communications!

In this chapter, a good percentage of my efforts will be spent demonstrating, from my experience, the approaches of multiple clinicians who are successful at convincing their patients to opt for the full-arch implant-supported prosthesis. By the conclusion of this chapter, you should have a good understanding of how such patients should be approached in your office.

Targeting your denture wearers first

This is a ripe market staring you right in the face, and you can't afford to ignore it. Any implant surgeon performing 500 or more implant placements per year, whom I am aware of, almost always performs an above-average number of full-arch, dental implant procedures.

I am reminded of one case in particular that affected a very well-experienced implantologist I met at an immediate-load course. His patient of 18 years got to a point where she could no longer tolerate her lower denture and apparently responded to an ad she saw on television, went in for a consult, and $24,000 later received a full-arch, fixed hybrid on four implants. She came back to this doctor's office approximately 3 months later, as instructed by the dental implant center, for her first cleaning.

The patient then ranted and raved about her new "implant bridge." She told this dentist that she felt like she had her life back and that this was the best money she'd spent on herself since buying her retirement Mercedes Benz 2 years prior. The doctor was extremely embarrassed by the fact that his then-denture patient hadn't talked to him first about dental implants. He also took issue with the dental implant center for "stealing his patient." I understand the part about being embarrassed, as he should have been. But this was no one's fault but his for having not seen or reached out to his patient since he last relined her denture more than 4 years ago.

Whether you only surgically place implants, only restore implants, or do both, if you don't consistently make it known to each and every one of your denture patients of record that you perform implant dentistry in your practice and are capable of delivering fixed-implant-supported teeth on the same day as surgery, you are making a very big mistake. In today's market, you will lose some of these patients to other practitioners who understand how to market their implant businesses and consequently miss out on the opportunity to transcend the quality of life for many individuals.

Here, we will focus on tactical marketing approaches designed to help your denture patients replace their outdated prostheses with full-arch, implant-supported prostheses. Whether it's a removable denture supported by four to six implants or a fixed-hybrid prosthesis supported by four, five, or six implants, part of your mission needs to be geared toward converting your denture-wearing patients into implant-supported prostheses—bottom line.

And when you begin to consistently and adequately present your denture patients with a dental implant-supported treatment plan, you will more frequently find the mandibular denture-wearing patient most eager to accept your treatment plan for obvious reasons.

Don't be afraid to make the most of this fact for the benefit of the patient. In no way, shape, or form is this unethical. Forget about what you think the patient can afford. Dental professionals tell me all the time, "My patients can't afford implants." So let me state it again: *Forget about what you think the patient can afford.* Your obligation is to inform your patient of the full-arch teeth replacement solutions that are far superior to a denture.

For starters, every one of your denture patients of record should routinely receive a courtesy letter from you as a basic follow-up, as demonstrated in Box 4.2. My recommendation is that you mail this letter to each of your denture patients three to four times per year. Additionally, every denture patient of record should also be on your target mailing list for your dental implant patient-education seminars. This is yet another reason it behooves you to offer these seminars each and every month, as discussed in Chapter 2.

Box 4.2 A quarterly letter as a follow-up to denture patients works well.

Denture patients keep in touch letter

Dear Denture Wearer [personalized],

I have decided to write you because it's been some time since we last saw you for treatment, and I wondered if all is well with your denture. When our denture patients stay away for more than a year, we've come to realize that it means they are so pleased with their denture that they don't feel a need to see us, or quite frankly, they have become frustrated with their denture and have literally given up on any viable solution to using it.

We hope you are pleased with your denture, but also realize there is a possibility that you have limited use, just based on the nature of a denture. In either case, it is still ideal to have your denture evaluated periodically.

As a courtesy, I would like to invite you in for a free evaluation. Simply give my office a call at (202) 222-2222, speak to Susie at the front desk, and let her know you'll need to come in for a complementary evaluation of your denture as soon as possible. I have already informed Susie that you might be calling and when you call she is to make room on the schedule for you.

Everyone should have the ability to eat, smile, and socialize with the confidence of stable teeth. Give us a call at your earliest convenience.

Sincerely,
Dr. John Lee

Face-to-face with the denture patient

When you begin to be face-to-face with your denture patients more frequently as a direct result of your concerted efforts, your verbal skills need to be in order. And I can't stress enough how key it is for you to avoid sugarcoating the patient's circumstances in your discussions. In Chapter 1, I discussed extensively the importance of showing *empathy*, not *sympathy*. This is vital with denture patients. Be compassionate and caring, but showing sympathy won't help the patient think about their resources.

Like Jack Webb said in *Dragnet*, and later imitated by Bruce Willis in *Die Hard II*, "Just the facts, ma'am." You need to get comfortable with giving your patients the facts. In no uncertain terms, tell the patient that bone loss is usually accelerated by an ill-fitting denture or that studies have shown denture-wearing patients take substantially more drugs (compared to individuals with a full capacity to chew their food) including higher rates of medication for gastrointestinal problems such as heartburn, stomach pain, or bloating (Misch & Misch, 1991). If the denture is loose, have the patient understand they need to replace it with dental implants while they still have enough bone to do so without requiring a major bone graft, if, in fact, this is the case.

Just because your denture patients aren't expressing chronic discomfort to you doesn't mean they aren't headed for a train wreck. An unsuspecting medical patient suddenly informed by the endocrinologist that she's showing signs of osteoporosis couldn't possibly know this to be a fact until it is brought to her attention by the physician. It is then incumbent upon the physician to create the sense of urgency for the patient, so steps can be taken to mitigate the problem. This is a commonsense expectation that all patients should place on their doctors.

A 5- or 10-year-old denture that is now ill fitting, I'm guessing, is probably an easily recognizable symptom of bone loss that can be verified with a panoramic X-ray. Your denture patients depend on you to inform them of the bone loss and to create a sense of urgency so that they can take steps to prevent the problem from getting worse. The only thing they know is that their denture isn't working for them anymore.

Why would you choose to reline or remake your patient's denture without first thoroughly educating them on the major underlying problem—bone loss? When patients have periodontal disease, they are informed that they will lose teeth, if appropriate action is not taken to manage the disease. Once patients lose their teeth, why don't more dentists tell patients they will lose jawbone if implants aren't placed? I have yet to be given a reasonable answer to either of these questions, by any dental professional.

If you, too, find it challenging to offer an acceptable answer to these questions, allow me to let you in on a secret. No person wants to lose bone. In fact, if every dentist were suddenly charged with educating their edentulous patients on the potential for jawbone loss and to compassionately inform them that dental implants are the best long-term solution to avoiding such a problem, the number of dental implant cases everywhere would increase dramatically, and the number of patients trading in their tissue-borne dentures for a full-arch, implant-supported prosthesis would skyrocket. Major implant companies would find it difficult to maintain adequate levels of inventory. That's how large the denture market is and how rapid the implant market would grow.

There are 48 million edentulous arches in the United States alone. You would only need a small percentage of these patients to accept treatment, many of whom would also opt for immediate-occlusal loading.

Immediate load/immediate function

As a clinician, you should want *immediate load* to be the surgical method by which your full-arch implant cases are administered. Immediate-load patients not only look forward to the destination, they also "appreciate the journey." The patient's journey is extremely important when it comes to marketing full-arch implant dentistry in your practice. And the easier you can make the journey for your full-arch implant patients, the more friends and family members they will refer. The opposite is also true. I know this to be factual based on multiple discussions with clinicians and an interesting random discussion I had with an implant patient.

I met a very nice 60-something-year-old implant recipient once at an Academy of Osseointegration convention. She happened to be an entrance guard to the exhibitor hall and understood that this was a dental convention. As we talked, I gathered that she had ultimately received a full-arch, fixed prosthesis. I asked her how she felt about her implant teeth, and she immediately replied, "I love them now because I can eat anything I want." But then she carried on about how dreadfully long the process was and how much she hated all the appointments and her loose-fitting (tissue-borne provisional) denture. As I continued to listen, it was obvious that, as she was going through the process, she believed that she had made a very bad decision. She went on to say, "For many months, I couldn't wear the denture to eat because it didn't help at all. I hated it."

Now, how many times do you think she's told that story to her friends and family members, who, by the way, are most likely candidates for dental implants also? She's enjoying the destination, but "hated the journey," and unfortunately, her journey is what she spent most of the time telling me about.

A patient's dreaded 4–6 month waiting period for the delivery of the final fixed-hybrid or zirconia prosthesis can be replaced with a far superior experience if they leave with a fixed-provisional prosthesis on the same day that the implants were placed. When this is the case, the patient can leave every appointment that follows, including impression-taking, face-bowl, smile-design, phonetics-observing, and bite-registration procedure, with a fixed-provisional prosthesis that they can appreciate and function with. The experience of a tissue-borne provisional implant patient, compared to an immediate-load patient, is like night and day.

One implant company might call it *TeethXpress®*, another might refer to it as *All-on-4®*, yet another has coined this protocol *RevitaliZe®*. These are all terms different companies trademark to classify their

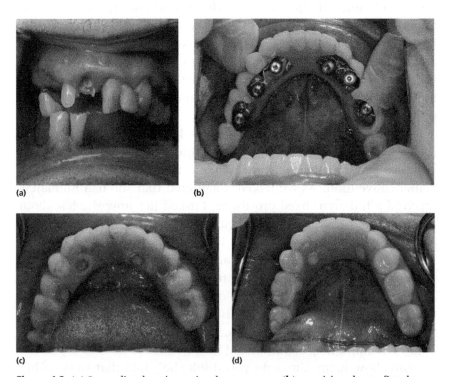

(a)   (b)

(c)   (d)

Figure 4.2 (**a**) Immediately prior to implant surgery, (**b**) provisional retrofitted to implants, (**c**) provisional fixed to implant abutments, and (**d**) final fixed prosthesis delivered in 3 months.

TeethXpress® is a registered trademark of BioHorizons. All-on-4® is a registered trademark of Nobel Biocare. RevitaliZe® is a registered trademark of Zimmer Dental.

full-arch, immediate-load protocol. Call it what you want, but what matters here is that you understand we are talking about marketing full-arch, immediate-occlusal loading, aka "immediate load," in very generic terms, because regardless of the implant system, the prosthetic protocols are quite similar (Figure 4.2).

Targeting removable partial denture and fixed partial denture patients for immediate load

Removable partial denture (RPD) and fixed partial denture (FPD) wearers are great targets for full-arch, immediate load. These are the patients who are not particularly pleased with the condition of their old and worn-down prostheses and the limitations these prostheses place on their quality of life. Obviously, I am not referring to the patients with one or two pontics, unless the rest of their teeth are severely infected with periodontal disease and the long-term prognosis is poor.

In my analysis, the most common reason why these patients continue to put up with poor esthetics or insufficient functionality is because they have never been given enough clinical rationale for replacing their RPD or FPD with dental implants. To a lesser degree, they are not aware of the possibilities of having the implants surgically placed and a full-arch implant-supported (provisional) prosthesis delivered all in the same day.

Most RPD–FPD patients who are ideal candidates for immediate load can barely come to grips with ever wearing a traditional, tissue-borne denture for any period of time, not even for 3–5 months, while their dental implants are left to osseointegrate and the final, fixed prosthesis is being fabricated. Immediate load is your fastest way to the hearts of this segment of the market. While the average practice is flooded with these patients, don't expect the typical patient to volunteer that they are a candidate for immediate load. They don't even know what immediate load is. Your practice has to present this solution in a compelling way.

Presenting the treatment plan for immediate load

I used to wonder why one dentist could present a full-arch, fixed-hybrid treatment plan to 10 patients and have 6 or 7 accept it, while another doctor, within the same city limits and socioeconomic environment, also presents 10 full-arch, fixed-hybrid treatment plans only to have one patient accept the proposed treatment plan option. This is no longer a mystery to me. I have worked with enough dentists now to know that such results are often on the opposite end of the pendulum, in large part, due to the confidence and verbal skills of the dentist and his or her staff.

You can use other marketing strategies to bring immediate-load candidates to your practice, but before you can ever hope to perform more immediate-load procedures, you must first be able to convince the patient to accept your treatment plan. Without being confident and having solid verbal communication skills to talk specifically about immediate load, a reasonable percentage of your patients will not agree to this procedure. Solid verbal skills involve the use of heartfelt communications to influence your patients to agree to a comprehensive full-arch, fixed-implant-supported prosthetic treatment plan.

With such patients, you must take your time to convince them that this is the absolute best option. It's not uncommon for the conversation to take an hour or more. Whatever it takes, you and your staff should be prepared to meet the demands.

The failing partial-denture: Post-op examination discussion

Here we will dissect the conversation of how an immediate load case presentation might go. I will cut in and out of the conversation to highlight critical points but pay particular attention to how the visual aids and verbal skills are used to help the patient appreciate the importance of moving forward with the proposed treatment plan. While I have spared you the small talk here, please bear in mind that there is a definite place for it.

We will assume the doctor intends to present the following patient with a full-arch, immediate load prosthesis as his best option. Keep in mind that these can sometimes be lengthy discussions, and in the following scripted example, I have tried to streamline the discussion as much as possible. But if you are not accustomed to routinely closing large, full-arch, implant-supported cases, please do not skip or skim through this section. It may not be the easiest read for you, but you should understand the type of dialogue that clinicians—who perform anywhere from 5 to 15 of such chases per month—have with their prospective implant patients. Let's get into it:

Dentist	Mrs. Smith, it's good meeting you today and thank you so very much for choosing to have us examine your partial and the condition of your oral health. And thank you as well, Mr. Smith, for being here with your wife today. [Allow Mr. Smith to respond, then carry on.] It's always best for the patient when the spouse understands what's causing the problems early on, so that you are both in the best position to make an informed decision based on the treatment options that I will put together and invite you both back to cover in detail.

Note here that the prospective implant patient's spouse is present. When it comes to acceptance of larger cases, the earlier you can get the spouse or significant other involved, the greater your chances are that the patient will ultimately accept your treatment plan.

In his book, *The Dentist's Unfair Advantage*, I like how *Big Case Marketing* founder and CEO, Dr. James McAnally, put it when he discusses the importance of having what he calls "The Decider" (the spouse or significant other) present at the treatment plan consultation appointment (McAnally, 2013). Dr. McAnally says, "That person is the second (and sometimes third) individual who has major input into financial decisions and whether a case goes forward.... In the majority of cases, when this individual is absent, what could have been a decision to correct a major dental problem will be pushed to the wayside simply because this individual was not at the appointment." Make sure you attempt to have the spouse involved as early as possible. To continue with the dialogue:

Dentist	Mrs. Smith, I know you have become very frustrated with your lower partial. According to my notes, you replaced your old partial denture with this partial denture about 3 years ago and have never been satisfied with it, and more recently, it has become very loose. And even after adjustments were made by your most recent dentist, you are still hardly able to eat with it since it moves quite a bit when you chew your food. Is this all accurate?

Mrs. Smith	Yes, that's right. The only thing I somewhat like about my partial is the way that it looks, so I wear it in public. Other than that, it's awful. I wish Dr. Jones was still practicing because when he originally made my partial, I never had all these problems. I've had nothing but problems ever since my last dentist made this partial. I never could use it.
Dentist	Mrs. Smith, I would agree that this partial does look good on you. It looks like your previous dentist did as good a job of designing this type of removable partial as most any dentist could have done, myself included. And if Dr. Jones were still practicing, my guess is that he'd probably tell you he couldn't do much better at this point, given the present condition of your jawbone.
Mrs. Smith	Well, what do you mean? Are you telling me that something's wrong with my jaw and there isn't any hope?
Dentist	I didn't say that; there is almost always a solution for a situation like yours. In fact, we successfully treat patients suffering from loose partials like yours every day. For patients in your condition, I strongly recommend dental implants. Are you familiar with dental implants?
Mrs. Smith	Yes, somewhat. But Dr. Thompson, I've heard that dental implants are very expensive. I just want to be able to eat and smile again. I don't think my insurance covers that. I can't afford dental implants.
Dentist	That all depends on what you consider "very expensive." I will tell you that these days, dental implants happen to be one of the most popular procedures we perform here, and most of my patients are working-class citizens. It does take a commitment, but you sound pretty committed to not living the rest of your life handicapped by a partial that won't stay in place or allow you to eat whatever food you want.

Please note the importance here of directing this dialogue with Mrs. Smith toward the fact that replacing her partial with another partial is not a viable solution. The other point worth making here is that "expensive" is a relative term. Some might consider implants to be expensive, but still find a way to pay for them, just as this hypothetical dentist is expecting his patient (Mrs. Smith) to become resourceful if she hopes to be happy with her teeth again.

In my experience, this is where most dentists begin to shy away from the objections. This is a very bad instinct. The dentist who routinely performs these procedures is prepared to answer these objections. In this case, she's only objecting because she doesn't know any better. Like Mrs. Smith, your patients count on you to make it clear for them. This next section covers some critical points worth making to the patient:

Dentist	In a moment, I'm going to have Lisa (the implant coordinator) show you a quick, 2-minute video that demonstrates exactly how missing teeth cause jawbone loss and how a partial denture like yours can do nothing to stop this bone loss and, in fact, causes damage to the remaining teeth.
Mrs. Smith	Dr. Thompson you keep saying "bone loss," what do you mean "bone loss"?
Dentist	Let me explain. [Using the mandible bone loss model to demonstrate, as seen in Figure 4.3.] You see this jaw with the teeth still in place?
Mrs. Smith	Yes.
Dentist	[Pointing to the edentulous mandible just to the right of it] Well, this jaw here is the same jaw as the one on the left, except the teeth have been removed. Now look at this jaw here [pointing to the jaw on the lower left]. Can you see that it's much smaller than the top two jaw models above it?
Mrs. Smith	Yeah, that's pretty easy to see. Why is that?
Dentist	Well, this is what happens over time in areas where there are no teeth in the mouth to stimulate the jawbone. Since receiving your original partial denture from Dr. Jones, you have suffered significant bone loss in areas where there are no teeth. Your jaw doesn't look like this anymore [pointing to the upper-right mandible with sufficient bone]. Now, your jaw looks much more like this beneath your partial [pointing to the third and fourth mandible with severe atrophy]. As a result, there is no bone left in these areas to help stabilize a partial denture. This will place even greater stress on two [abutment teeth] of your remaining five teeth, and that's not enough to keep a partial stable when you talk and eat.
Mrs. Smith	My jawbone looks like this because I wear a partial? [She's pointing to the fourth mandible.]
Dentist	In part, yes! The biggest reason you have lost significant bone and muscle mass is because when your teeth were removed, there was no longer any root structure anchored in your jawbone, and without the roots of your teeth, over the years your jawbone has melted away. Teeth help to keep your jawbone from shrinking.
Mrs. Smith	Well now, what the hell do I do since I've loss so much bone?

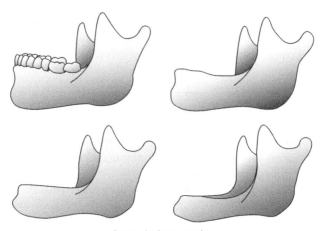

Progressive bone atrophy

Figure 4.3 Use mandible bone-loss model to demonstrate progressive jawbone atrophy to edentulous patients.

Now, you have Mrs. Smith's attention. She is very open to learning more. Besides, no one has taken the time to explain it to her this way in the past. Consequently, money is less of an issue, and dental insurance is not her biggest concern at this moment. She's already thinking out loud, "How do I fix this problem now?" And though her husband, Thomas, has kept quiet, he too is wondering how his wife can be helped.

Dentist	We've successfully treated several people with worse conditions than yours, but doing so requires replacing the roots of your missing teeth with artificial roots, also known as dental implants. First of all, we have to stop the bone loss in its tracks. Dental implants are your best option for this. Dental implants will also give us the ability to stabilize your teeth, even better than the original partial that you liked. You will be able to chew and grind your food better than you have in years—I can assure you of this. But you have to be willing to listen with an open mind to the dental implant option—financially and otherwise—because it's our most successful option to solving your problem.
Mrs. Smith	I'm willing to listen because honestly I don't even enjoy going out to dinner anymore. It's too embarrassing.
Dentist	What do you mean? Tell me why it's embarrassing for you to eat out....

Mrs. Smith	I can't chew my food well with my partial denture in. Food gets under it and then it gets loose. So I have to take it out just to chew my food. But when I take it out, my mouth looks horrible, and everyone at the table can see how many missing teeth I have when I talk. So, I find myself talking and smiling as little as possible when I go out to dinner. But then everyone knows how much I like to talk, so they start asking me, "What's wrong?" I hate it.
Dentist	Mrs. Smith, this is a common problem that many patients in your situation deal with every day. At your next appointment, I will show you how your problem can be solved quickly. For now, I'm going to have you see Lisa in the consultation room. She'll share more information with you on dental implants and answer any basic questions you might have. Lisa will then get you and Mr. Smith both scheduled to come back and see me for a [free] consultation so that I can recommend a treatment plan that will give you nice-looking teeth that allow you to eat better than you have in years. Would that be okay?
Mrs. Smith	Yes, that sounds good. Thank you Dr. Thompson.

Now, your patient will meet briefly with your implant coordinator who has already queued up the bone-loss, partial denture, and basic dental implant animations. While your very competent auxiliary staff member presents the video, sings your praises, and answers the more general questions your prospective implant patient might not have asked you, you're off to see your next patient.

Consultation with the immediate-load candidate

Your immediate-load candidate should be invited to come back for a free consultation no longer than 1 week later. It is imperative that you either block out space for implant consultations or find a way to fit in a patient—like Mrs. Smith—no later than 1 week from the date of her examination. Your patient will never be more motivated to move forward with your dental implant treatment plan than during the first few days following your examination.

Now, let's fast forward to the following week where Mrs. Smith is back in for her consultation. If you are wisely using 3D images from a CBCT machine, sharing these images with your patients to highlight conditions specific to the patient's case can be very helpful. Just be sure that you have virtually positioned the implants in your CBCT-generated images, as this will give the patient a stronger sense of what will be required to achieve the end goal.

That said, particularly in your larger cases, the influence a very good animation can have on an implant prospect is priceless. Your patients need to be able to visualize the end result. I often say CT scans are to clinicians what dental implant animations are to patients.

Therefore, in this scenario of having Mr. and Mrs. Smith back for her consultation, we will pull out a fixed and removable model. We will also need to have our personalized, animated dental implant software queued up. Your conversation should pick up something like this:

Dentist	Mrs. Smith, thank you for choosing to come back for your consultation. And thank you as well, Mr. Smith, for being here in support of your wife once again. Mrs. Smith, at your last visit, if you recall, we spent a great deal of time discussing your condition. My number one priority today is to educate you both on Mrs. Smith's options so that you are best positioned to make an informed decision. Fair enough?
Mrs. Smith	Yes.
Dentist	I know you have become very frustrated with your lower partial. You've had this partial denture for 3 years and have never really been satisfied with it, and more recently, it has become very loose, and even after adjustments, you are still hardly able to eat with it since it moves quite a bit when you chew your food. I gathered that this upsets you quite a bit because you enjoy "breaking bread" with friends and family, but can't really enjoy yourself to the fullest because your teeth don't allow you to eat and talk comfortably in social settings. Is this all accurate?
Mrs. Smith	Yes, that's correct.
Dentist	Mrs. Smith, at your last visit, Lisa showed you an animated video of exactly how missing teeth lead to bone loss and how dental implants work. This should give you a better picture of how you arrived to this point of bone loss and the purpose of dental implants. I have two dental implant models that I will use to demonstrate with for starters. In a situation like yours where you have only five [mandibular] remaining teeth, for better functionality and looks, I recommend removing these few teeth and giving you a full set of new teeth that are supported by four to five dental

	implants. The first model is what we call a "removable" implant overdenture. [Hand the patient the Removable Overdenture Locator® model (see Figure 4.4).] Mrs. Smith, these teeth are held in place by four dental implants. I want you to try removing these teeth from the implants it's attached to … Not so easy, is it?
Mrs. Smith	No, I can hardly take it off at all. [Have the significant other attempt to do so as well.] But why can't you leave my teeth there and place dental implants in the spaces of the missing teeth?
Dentist	We can do that, but to keep your remaining teeth in will require placing more implants, at least six to seven. To do it right will require adequate bone grafting that will cause your treatment to take twice as long, and add to the overall cost, and I've tried very hard to keep your cost down. Additionally, these five teeth [using the patient's cast] are so badly diseased that they are exuding puss. To save them will require extensive periodontal surgery, and even then I can't be confident that they will last you much longer. Again, if we take these diseased teeth out, we will only need to place four to five implants to support a complete set of teeth like what you see on these two models.

Now is a great time to show Mrs. Smith (and Mr. Smith) a personalized, animated video that will visually walk them through the process she can expect. No need to go into extensive detail even at this point, but you do want to give them a visual of how this process will transpire. This video animation should be kept under 1 minute when

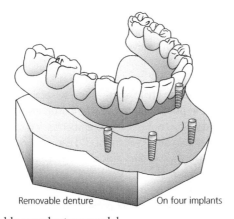

Removable denture   On four implants

Figure 4.4 Removable overdenture model.

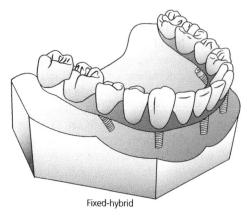

Fixed-hybrid

Figure 4.5 Fixed-hybrid model with four, five, or six implants.

possible. You'll also need a fixed-hybrid model to describe immediate load (see Figure 4.5):

Dentist	You have great questions, Mrs. Smith, and this is probably a good time to show you exactly how we can best manage your case from start to finish. [Press "play" to your queued-up video animation and describe the protocol as need be.] Mrs. Smith, as you can see, these are the exact teeth you have remaining. [Animation shows teeth being removed.] As you see, we will remove these teeth, level your underlying bone, and insert the implants. The full set of teeth is then bolted down to the implants—just as you see here—so that by the time you leave, you have your implants and a new set of teeth attached to the implants.
Mrs. Smith	This is all done in one visit?
Dentist	That is correct. Essentially, this is the protocol my team and I will take to satisfy your case. Before you know it, you would have regained your ability to enjoy a nice vegetable salad and a tender steak out in public without any embarrassment whatsoever.
Mrs. Smith	Yes. That's why I'm here. It's so embarrassing to eat in public, and I'm tired of avoiding certain foods I can no longer chew very well.
Dentist	Mrs. Smith, the second model is what we call a fixed-implant bridge because like natural teeth, these teeth are designed to remain in place, permanently. This is the scenario I just demonstrated in the video. Most patients prefer *fixed* because it never

comes out except when you visit us for a professional cleaning. With this option, we have the flexibility to make the teeth look more natural and less like a denture as with the *removable* example, and as you can see, these fixed teeth are more con- toured since it doesn't require as much acrylic as the *removable* prosthesis. The other advantage to the *fixed* prosthesis is that on the day that we place your implants, we can immediately lock your teeth in place, as described in the video. We call this "immediate load" because it allows you to go out and enjoy a soft diet on your implant teeth "immediately" following your surgery.

Mrs. Smith   Why can't I eat immediately on my implants with this [removable] option?

Dentist   Great question. Anytime you have a removable prosthesis like this one [*removable model*], you must wait 3–6 months for the implants to heal before we can attach the implants to the teeth. If we connect a removable prosthesis to the implants before they heal, the implants will fail since the removable teeth are meant to snap in and out. Snapping teeth in and out on implants that haven't fully healed in your bone is what will cause them to fail. For that 3–6-month period, your denture will rest on your gums while your implants heal beneath your gums. And in your case, where you have already suffered significant bone loss, wearing a full denture on top of your gums for 3–6 months might be quite annoying if it doesn't stay in place. With the *fixed* option, the teeth are locked in place from day one. You can eat in public and smile freely and know that your teeth won't move. Make sense?

Mrs. Smith   Yes. I just wonder what it will cost me to have implants and teeth like these and how long it will take. I know I have good insurance. Will my insurance cover any of this?

We're in a good place right now. The patient and the significant other are both engaged. The patient is motivated and has demon- strated that she wants this. And we have given the patient options.

The dentist should be encouraged that the patient has expressed interest in what this will all cost her. This is not a time to shy away from the cost or to sympathize with the patient if she makes it seem impossible to come up with the money for something she now desires to have badly. The patient needs to feel like she is in the company of so many others who looked deeply into their resources to find a way to pay for this treatment.

Another point worth making here is that when you are dealing with a case of this size and scope, it behooves you to put away your pride and help the patient maximize their dental benefits, even if you are fee-for-service. The patient doesn't know that dental insurance is mostly senseless, and now is not the time to get into a philosophical discussion about it. Obviously, stay within the law, and look for every scenario possible to help your patient maximize the benefits in a full-arch implant case such as this.

Now that we are ready to talk finances, and as we seek a buy-in from the spouse, it's time to address him far more directly. Also at this point, if you have a well-trained implant coordinator or financial coordinator who has been taught to discuss the clinical aspects of implant dentistry and is capable of discussing larger dollar amounts and proficiently working out payment terms, this is a good time to bring that person into the fold while you carry on with your day:

Dentist   Mrs. Smith, my staff is very good at helping our patients get the most from their benefits. But I have to tell you, patients that opt for dental implants generally see this as an investment in their health and quality of life because most end up financing the bulk of this expense in some way. The first option [pointing to the *removable model*] is less expensive at about $14,000 total. Your second option certainly has its advantages over the first, as we've discussed [pointing to the *fixed-hybrid model*]. This option is closer to $25,000. It's a bigger financial commitment but clearly the best solution for your condition.

You remember my implant coordinator, Lisa.... Lisa is far more efficient at discussing finances and walking you though your payment options than I could ever hope to be. So at this point, I will have her to take care of you if that's ok. She knows that I will be right up the hall if you should need me to answer any more questions for you. Otherwise, you are in great hands. Again, thank you Mr. and Mrs. Smith for your time, and I hope we can move forward with treatment real soon. Thank you Lisa, please take care of these good folks for me!

Implant Coordinator (LISA)	Thank you Dr. Thompson. I will do just that.... Mr. and Mrs. Smith it's good to see you again.... We can talk finances shortly, and I'll be sure to present to you all the options, but may I first ask you which option do you prefer, the fixed or the removable option?
Mrs. Smith	I like the option of having teeth that don't have to come out. But can you explain why that option cost so much more?
Implant Coordinator (LISA)	Certainly. Unlike the *removable*, your teeth will be *locked* in place just like natural teeth, and because they're locked in place everything we do on our end, from the amount of appointments, to the laboratory materials, to the required dental implant parts, everything is more expensive. Obviously, in order for us to provide this amazing service, we have to charge a higher fee so that the teeth will look, function, and feel more like your natural teeth. At $25,000, this option is more expensive, but I encourage it because patients are more satisfied with it. You have fixed bridgework on day 1. The removable also functions very well once the implants are healed 3–6 months later. But quite frankly, it's less expensive because it's less costly to manufacture since it snaps in and out.
Mrs. Smith	Obviously, the fixed teeth would be my first choice, too, but I certainly didn't intend to spend some $25,000 for teeth, and we don't have that kind of money sitting around.
Implant Coordinator (LISA)	I completely understand Mrs. Smith. If you prefer the second option, I can tell you that most of our patients don't have this money sitting in the bank, and so like any worthwhile investment, they end up financing the better part of it. You might remember Mrs. Philips from the patient seminar you attended a couple weeks ago when she gave a testimonial about her dental implant teeth? She drives a school bus. She took out a bank loan to cover most of her procedure. Would you and Mr. Smith consider financing this?
Mrs. Smith	I guess I could finance it, but I'm not sure if I'd be approved for that amount.

Implant Coordinator (LISA)	Well, let's look at what you would actually need to finance first. I've researched your insurance plan and based on the procedures you will require, I'm certain we can help you maximize your total dental benefits at $1,000, so now we're down to $24,000. What can you afford to pay in cash?
Mrs. Smith	I was prepared to pay up to $5,000 for a new set of teeth.
Implant Coordinator (LISA)	Okay, good. Now, we're basically looking at $19,000. If you're able to finance the $19,000 at a relatively low interest rate, you can get your payments down to around $400 per month. We work with a couple different medical financing companies. They offer interest-free or low-interest-rate financing. Other patients prefer to go through their bank or credit union. Would the two of you consider either of these options?
Mrs. Smith	Well, what do you think Thomas [her spouse]?
Mr. Smith (Spouse)	Well, if this is what it will require to get you taken care of, I think you should do it. I think we should just go through our bank and finance the difference. I'm sure we can get a reasonable interest rate. When can she get started once we've secured the finances?
Implant Coordinator (LISA)	Mr. Smith, the surgeon we work with reserves Friday mornings for these types of procedures. I'll verify with his office that he has a space for you as early as next week on Friday. He and Dr. Thompson will perform this procedure together as a team at his office. This will give you time to speak with your bank. If we can have you place your $5000 down today, we can take impressions before you leave today so that we can secure the provisional teeth we'll need to attach to your implants at the time of your surgery next week.

This conversation demonstrates that convincing your patients to opt for premium cases such as full-arch, immediate load requires the use of solid marketing efforts to attract such patients in need and good visual aids and verbal skills necessary to achieve case acceptance. This is a must. If the patient would have opted for the less expensive implant-supported removable prosthesis, or even a traditional tissue-borne denture, either would have been completely acceptable as well. It is always the patient's choice based on their priorities and what they can afford. In this example, what is important from the provider's standpoint is that the conversation took place under the most compelling and compassionate conditions possible.

Doctors that are successful in full-arch implant dentistry, which I know personally, are consistent in their efforts when it comes to patient communication. These doctors exercise similar patient communications characteristics, over and over again. Perhaps one of the most common characteristics is the fact that they don't allow their preconceived notions to get in the way of what is presented to the patient.

Making financial arrangements

The only thing left to do now is to agree on the financial arrangements and to get the patient scheduled for treatment. It's important you understand that you, the dentist, should never shy away from disclosing your fees. But once you have put the fee out there and have discussed it freely, it's ideal to bring a capable, confident staff member in to sort out the details and to make final arrangements for collection.

Once the patient has agreed in principle to treatment, this is the time to have a staff member who is comfortable with discussing large sums of money to intersect and solidify the financial agreement. If that staff member is confident, compassionate, and capable of making financial arrangements on full-arch cases that can range as high as $25,000, $50,000, or $75,000, as invaluable as such a person may be, never assume they can maintain their success rate without you first doing your part to thoroughly help the patient appreciate the clinical solutions to their problems.

In the aforementioned demonstration, the patient has already made it clear that she has $5,000. Don't be cavalier about it. Secure this $5,000 on that same day if possible. This will go a long ways in having the patient commit. I have seen the money collected in different ways, but I generally advise collecting one- to two-thirds down if possible and the final one-third shortly before delivering the final prosthesis. That said, there are multiple successful ways of making financial arrangements with the patient. The final payment can be made in one or two visits prior to the delivery of the final prosthesis.

Establish goals for immediate-load production

Money cannot be your primary motivation for performing full-arch immediate load. If money becomes your primary reason for offering this service, it will come across to your patient, dictate the way you design your treatment plan (so that you may cut costs in every way), and therefore affect the quality of care you provide. With that said, full-arch immediate load is a tremendous service to any patient in need, and you should never feel guilty about earning a very attractive fee for your services.

To consistently increase the number of immediate load cases you perform each month and year, you must establish goals. Be realistic in setting your goals. If you have yet to perform an immediate load case, don't assume in the first month you will perform four or five arches simply because you know you have the cases available and the immediate load course you recently attended has you feeling invincible. Motivation is good, in fact, you won't perform very many of these cases without motivation. But anyone I know that consistently performs this procedure and performs it well has gradually arrived at that point.

Getting your first couple of cases behind you is key. Once you have done so and feel comfortable with the protocol, the lab tech support, surgical specialist, or restorative doctor, you can be confident that it is time to set meaningful goals and press forward.

A total fee in the vicinity of $25,000 to the patient for a full-arch immediate load procedure, definitively restored with a CAD/CAM metal framework, wrapped in acrylic, is commonplace in many markets around the United States. To determine your portion of the total fee, you will need to work the numbers out with the clinical members of your team based on each of your respective surgical and restorative costs. Offer a more esthetic solution such as full zirconia bridges or framework designed for individual e.max™ crowns, for example, and your patient should expect to pay a higher fee.

For simplicity, as seen in Figure 4.6, at $25,000 per arch, the numbers can escalate rapidly. Just five cases in 1 month can represent $125,000 in immediate load procedures. Clear ten arches in a month and between you and your team, that's $250,000 in production from immediate load, fixed-implant procedures. Maybe your goal is simply to average 1 per month or 12 inside of a year. What's most important is that you (and your team) establish a goal for how many patients

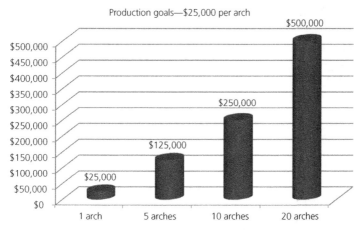

Figure 4.6 Annual goals for number of full-arch cases is critical to success.

you would like to provide this service to each month, and use the principles and tactical approaches found in this book to reach those goals. You can do it!

Summary

Whether it's removable or fixed, full-arch implant-supported prostheses offers tremendous value to most any patient in need. The key is to never prejudge the patient. Deliver your message to every prospective full-arch patient as if you know the patient has the resources to pay for your proposed treatment plan. Your obligation is to help each full-arch implant candidate understand their afflictions in the most empathetic and compelling way possible and to offer comprehensive options so that they can make informed decisions on solutions to their problems. An implant coordinator or administrative staff member who has a comprehensive knowledge of implant dentistry and is comfortable with discussing full-arch cases and collecting high dollar amounts can be a significant asset to case acceptance.

The literature has proven immediate load to be highly successful, in the high 97 percentage range. Learn how to perform this procedure well. Make use of effective visual aids and verbal skills when presenting this option to your patients, and your case acceptance for this procedure will improve significantly.

CHAPTER 5

Implant marketing for the surgical specialist

Yes, times have changed. Gone are the days where an oral surgeon and periodontist are virtually the only dental professionals trained and skilled enough to perform dental implant surgery. More restorative dentists are being taught to perform dental implant surgery, some as early as dental school. But so what! There are far more dental implant opportunities available for every clinician, none more so than for the surgical specialist.

I wish I could tell you that if you don't agree with most of what you will read in this chapter and book, to just do nothing at all to enhance your marketing strategy, and everything will remain the same for you. But to offer such poor advice would be irresponsible and way off the mark. In fact, I am confident that maintaining the status quo will assuredly cause your implant business to follow a downward trend in the coming years. But wouldn't this be in line with every other aspect of business?

One of the most profound short stories apropos to the ways of business is *Who Moved My Cheese*, by Spenser Johnson, MD. In this lighthearted fable (of two little people named Hem and Haw and two mice named Sniff and Scurry), the four characters each started their daily journey with a similar set of circumstances and contentedly helped themselves to what seemed to be an endless supply of cheese. Until one day, it suddenly seemed the cheese had been moved. As the story concludes, it turns out that those quickest to adapt to change and seek a new supply of cheese

Marketing Implant Dentistry: Attract and Influence Patients to Accept Your Dental Implant Treatment Plan, First Edition. Marcus Hines.
© 2016 John Wiley & Sons, Inc. Published 2016 by John Wiley & Sons, Inc.

elsewhere eventually found their new supply and benefited the most. And the individual most reluctant to adapt and look for cheese elsewhere paid a much higher price, suffered, and ultimately perished.

Truth is, this is how business has always worked. No matter the industry, the "cheese" is always being moved. It is how we evolve and win in business and in society.

Automobile manufacturers are clearly concerned with the success of the Tesla Model S. Not only is this electric car good looking, but it requires no gasoline, has zero emissions, and is sold exclusively over the Internet—no dealership required. Taxicab drivers are forced to compete with an innovative company called Uber, which empowers its patrons to request a driver through the use of a smartphone app.

Even illegal drug dealers distributing marijuana can't be too complacent these days. Washington State's tax revenues from legal pot sales is nothing to laugh at. And since Colorado legalized marijuana for recreational use in January 2014, according to the Colorado Department of Revenue, their state had generated $29.8 million in tax revenues for the first half of the year (Associated-Press, 2014). I am not condoning the use of marijuana, but some reports estimate that for every pot dispensary opening, approximately ten illegal drug dealers will go out of business. Even the criminal minded must be in constant pursuit of new *cheese*!

Who moved my *implant*?

Like the cheese in the fable, do you sometimes feel that someone is moving your *implants*? If so, you're probably right. The bigger question is: What will you do about it? As a specialist, the sooner you adopt new and diverse ways of attracting implant patients, the better off you and the general public will be.

Consider the approach an increasingly popular dental implant center franchise has taken. By all accounts, these are specialty practices comprised of oral surgeons and prosthodontists. Their business model is not primarily geared around professional referrals, as with tradition. They go direct to the consumer. In fact, they spend tens of thousands of dollars each month going direct to consumer.

I love one of their television advertisements that presents a 50-something-year-old gentleman who expressed the poor condition his natural teeth were in. He went on to offer up a convincing testimonial about his wonderful experience of receiving implant-supported teeth through this particular dental implant center. The backdrop of this ad happened to be at his place of business: an auto repair shop. The message to the viewer is clear—if a respectable auto mechanic can afford dental implants, so can you. Brilliant!

As successful as this dental implant franchise's business model may be today, rest assured that their "cheese" will eventually be moved as well, and if it is to continue to thrive, looking for other sources of dental implant patients will be required, eventually.

The same is true of your specialty implant practice. There is no better time than the present to realize exponential growth. The patients are more plentiful than ever and enough of them can afford what you have to offer. Your challenge is whether or not you can envision the growth of your implant business through a different set of lenses. Albert Einstein said, "We cannot solve our problems with the same level of thinking that created them."

If you are willing to market your specialty practice through a different paradigm, as I will challenge you to do so in this chapter and in this book, you will position yourself to place far more implants than you have in the recent past. For now, let's begin with your professional relationships.

Meeting the needs of the restorative doctor

Professional referrals are no doubt familiar ground to any surgical specialist. There are several approaches any surgical specialist can take to improve his or her strategies on targeting the restorative doctor for more and better dental implant patient referrals.

Provide restorative parts

Providing your referring dentists with impression copings and laboratory analogs, in many instances, can be the determining factor for whether or not the next implant case is referred to you or your counterpart. Before complaining about how much this will all cost you, consider what it will cost if you unknowingly lose implant referrals to your competing specialists that wisely provide restorative parts while you don't. Assuming you charge a $2,000 surgical fee for each implant placed, losing just 20 implants in a year's time, between two referral sources, represents a $40,000 hit to your practice. Multiply this surgical fee by four accounts over a 5-year period, and at a $200,000 hit to your practice, the numbers can get ugly real fast.

In today's competitive environment, you need as many advantages working in your favor as possible. Dr. Ramin Azghandi, a Germantown, MD, periodontist, has provided his referring dentists with impression copings, laboratory analogs, and abutments for years. When you can help your referral sources appreciate that they are more profitable when they refer implant cases to you, you have given them one more reason to push the patient in your direction.

Clearly, there is a financial cost associated with this effort. But any surgical specialist that does this understands that the cost of giving away free parts pales in comparison to the monetary value that is a definite by-product of providing such parts.

If you choose to provide restorative parts, you will also want to understand the dentist's preferences. Some restorative doctors prefer closed-tray impression copings, while many prosthodontists insist on using an open-tray technique. The easier you make this process, the more your referring doctors will rely on you for future cases, especially when one of their patient's is treated by a different specialist and they are left to navigate their way through the restorative process all alone. It is during these moments when your referring dentists will appreciate you the most. Fortunately, this is an expandable effort that can be managed by your implant coordinator.

Superior professional and patient communications/ correspondences

If you view every dental implant patient referral as a gift and a vote of confidence in your specialty surgical skills, and you should, it makes all the sense in the world to thoroughly explore the wishes of the referring doctor, communicate your findings to the referring doctor, and openly share your recommendations to the referring doctor. Just as you spend time interviewing the patient, you need to make an effort to speak with the doctor prior to, during, and following treatment. This is to be sure that you (the specialist), the dentist, and the patient are all on one accord.

In my experience, there are certain specialists who understand the dynamics of professional and patient communications better than most. Dr. Rebecca Wagner, a periodontist practicing in Chambersburg, PA, is exceptionally detailed in her follow-up correspondence to her referring doctors. She understands that little frustrates a referring doctor more than not being informed on the details of implant placement until after the fact. Dr. Wagner says, "I send detailed communications to doctors via my *consult report letter* [following exam/ treatment plan], a *postsurgical implant letter* [following implant surgery], and a *resume letter* [following confirmation of osseointegration]."

Figure 5.1 is an example of how Dr. Wagner's postsurgical implant letter reads. As an implant representative, I have read hundreds of

Wagner Centre at CVDC

Rebecca L. Wagner, DDS, MS
Diplomate, American Board of Periodontology
Fellow, International Congress of Oral Implantologists

Implants, Periodontics & Oral Medicine

October 9, 2014

Re: Susan J.

Dear Dr. Landon,

A single stage implant surgery was completed for our mutual patient Susan J. The implant was placed in good position and healing collar was also placed. The type of Biohorizons Laser Lok implant placed as well as other surgical information is detailed below. Susan tolerated the procedure quite well. Please plan to begin the restorative phase anytime.

Please don't hesitate to contact our office with any questions.

Site	Diameter	Platform	Length	Healing collar	Tissue Height
#7	3.0mm	3mm	12mm	TP3HA3	2mm
#10	3.0mm	3mm	12mm	TP3HA3	2mm

Sincerely

Rebecca L Wagner

Rebecca L. Wagner, D.D.S., M.S.

Comments: Enclosed: D-PA, Please order Transfer coping from Biohorizons for 3.0 Implant.

**The item number for the 3.0 Indirect Scoop Coping is #TP3ISC

If you have any questions please contact us or our Biohorizons Representative Marcus Hines at 1-301-785-8424.

99 St. Paul Drive • Chambersburg, PA 17201
717.263.0606 Tel • 717.264.4346 Fax • drwagner@wagnerctr.com

Figure 5.1 Example of detailed postsurgical follow-up letter.

postimplant surgery letters, and most of these letters simply do not include enough restorative-driven information. In this letter, note that the implant diameters and lengths are listed on her report. More importantly, Dr. Wagner also listed restorative platforms and soft tissue heights. To the dentist, knowing the restorative platform(s) is just as critical as it is for the surgical specialist to know the implant diameter and length, and when she does not provide restorative components, she lists the "item number" for the office to order. Even the soft tissue thickness is included for each implant. This comes in handy in cases where the dentist prefers to use a prefabricated/stock abutment and is absolutely vital in cases where Locator® overdenture abutments or multiunit abutments will be used in a full-arch restoration.

Dr. Wagner will tell you that much of her ability to establish a rapidly growing Chambersburg, PA, periodontal and implant practice from scratch has much to do with the establishment of systems and comprehensive professional and patient communications. She says, "I make it a point to meet with each of my implant referral sources individually on a quarterly or semiannual basis. They know I am available via e-mail, text messaging, or by phone whenever they need me. I offer to train their staff members on the rationale of implant dentistry, and I provide lunch and continuing education credits in the process. When their patients are under my care, I look for ways to genuinely complement the referring doctor, and each patient is given my cell number and my e-mail so that they can communicate with me at any time."

Sharing case reports with restorative doctors

One of the more common methods specialists tend to use to help elevate the clinical thought process and to stay in front of their surrounding restorative doctors is to host restorative-driven study group meetings. Others use monthly or quarterly newsletter to keep in touch. Both methods can serve their purposes well.

Another method I would have you consider for its efficacy is the sharing of case reports, white papers, studies, and so on with your surrounding restorative community. There are plenty of good implant case reports in industry journals such as the *Compendium*, *Implant Dentistry*, *Dentistry Today*, and the like.

Once you have located a dental implant-related article that you find fascinating, you must then read the article, in its entirety, followed by summarizing it (on your letterhead) in as few as two paragraphs followed by sending a copy of the article to your area restorative doctors.

As with the example in Box 5.1, this letter is not intended to be long. Rest assured that most of the doctors will not read the article in detail, but as long as you avoid making it long and drawn out, they will read your letter.

Because you have a captive audience, your goal is to achieve two primary objectives with the first being to maintain a constant respectable presence with your targeted audience. Mailing relevant case reports, studies, and articles four to six times a year will help you to achieve this goal. Your second goal here is to make an earnest effort at elevating the level of consciousness with restorative doctors in your area.

Box 5.1 Example of summarized letter to be included with case report.

Case report summary letter

Dear Dr. [personalize],

Multiple studies have shown that conventional denture-wearing patients avoid many coarse/hard foods including raw vegetables, meats, and fruits for the reason that these food types are difficult to chew. Consequently, major sources of vitamins, minerals, protein, and fiber are sacrificed.

For your review, I have enclosed a report titled *The Effects of Mandibular Two-Implant Overdentures on Nutrition in Elderly Edentulous Individuals*. The research in this report compared the health of conventional overdenture wearers with implant-supported overdenture wearers.

As explained in this report, conventional denture wearers were found to suffer from considerably low levels of *serum albumin*. Low levels of serum albumin are associated with higher rates of cancer, cardiovascular disease, and mortality. Conversely, patients who had their denture held in place by at least two dental implants demonstrated higher levels of serum albumin, largely due to their increased food choices and significantly improved chewing ability.

Denture patients make better choices about their oral health when they understand the overall health-related benefits of receiving dental implants. We encourage you to share the findings presented in this report with your staff and your patients.

If we can be of any assistance to you and your patients, please do not hesitate to call on us.

Sincerely,
Dr. Surgical Specialist

This process is simple and when applied over a period of at least 1–2 years, it works like a charm at maintaining a presence as well as educating and garnering respect. You will also begin to open your eyes to the clinical possibilities as you begin to review and summarize more and more case reports.

Edentulous patient implant study group

Before we get into exactly what an edentulous implant study group is and how it works, consider some basic statistics first. There are more than 30 million adults in the United States alone who are edentulous in at least one arch. Thirty million! The percentage of edentulism is decreasing, but people are living longer, and the adult population is rising so rapidly that individuals in need of one or two dentures are estimated to increase from 33.6 million back in 1991 to 37.9 million adults by the year 2020 (Douglass, Shih and Ostry, 2002).

But if you are the typical periodontist who generally does not receive the mostly edentulous or fully edentulous patient referral for implants, what do you do? You do what Hagerstown, MD-based periodontist Dr. Fred Bye did and create a learning environment by which general dentists can develop a better understanding of how to collaborate with you and use best practices to treat such patients with implants.

I watched Dr. Bye grow his implant business exponentially over the course of a 24-month period in large part due to his idea to form an edentulous study group. Here's how he explains it:

At times, I felt like I was all dressed up with nowhere to go. I had trained under some of the foremost respected clinicians, surgically and restoratively, but my implant business still was not as busy as I needed it to be. After doing the numbers it just made sense to start an edentulous patient club. I felt that if I handpicked 20 dentists and required each doctor to bring a minimum of two cases each year, the group would serve its mission of rehabilitating more edentulous patients with implant prosthetics. Dentists who had previously referred cases that only required one or two implants were suddenly referring two- and three-full-arch, implant cases each year. Our dental implant business grew almost exponentially upon establishing the implant study club. You could see the confidence in these doctors grow overnight and I couldn't be more pleased with the results of these study club meetings.

I am a very big fan of the surgical specialist running an edentulous dental implant study group. It's niche, there is a market for it, and not everyone is doing it. This is not a "study group" in the general sense of the term where you open the meeting up for all dentists to attend; they eat your steak dinner, drink your wine, nod off, wake up, and ask, "Where do I sign for my continuing education credits?" Such a study group has its place from a social and networking standpoint, but this isn't the purpose of this meeting.

An edentulous study group is designed to target the dentist who desires to learn more about restoring full-arch, dental implant-supported prostheses. The members of this edentulous study group recognize the value in engaging and sharing their experiences and their perspectives with all members of the group so that everyone learns. As a rule, there are no egos, no renowned speakers flying in to give presentations where only their cases are presented, yet little to no dialogue is offered.

You, the specialist, can be the only star in this show, but it is important that you also check your ego at the door, too. Regardless of how much you know or how elevated your experience, any sign of arrogance or appearing to be condescending in such a group setting and you are dead in the water.

Edentulous study group members must submit cases

This group is about learning and doing, and in order to learn, you must do. Members of this edentulous study group should know that they are expected to commit to a minimum of two full-arch, implant-supported cases each year. Because the membership is dependent on studying multiple cases to learn from, if certain members are not submitting cases, in many ways, they are keeping the group back from achieving its primary mission, which is to grow the skill set in full-arch, implant-supported reconstruction.

By the way, every restorative doctor has several patients in his or her practice that are willing to accept a treatment plan for a full-arch, implant-supported prosthesis, assuming the treatment plan is presented in the right way. As long as your referring doctors don't understand how to restore these full arches, they will tell you, "My patients can't afford it." When your restorative doctors understand how to restore these cases and witness successful cases that their colleagues have restored, the confidence to treatment plan, and present full-arch implant-supported cases will soon follow.

The two patients per dentist are expected to be sent to your office for a CBCT scan, examination, and dental implant treatment plan. The dentist and you, the specialist, will then devise a treatment plan for the case together, and when the time comes for you, the specialist, to present this case before all members of the study group, the referring dentist will be called on to tell the patient's story and share any restorative pearls of wisdom before the other group members.

I watched Dr. Bye present several treatment plans, including virtual implant positions, required bone grafting and ridge augmentations, and postsurgical images, followed by his encouragement of the referring dentist to chime in and discuss the restorative steps they took to arrive at the final prosthetic delivery. There is a natural synergistic energy in the room as the surgical specialist and referring dentist team up to walk through each of these cases. Naturally, other dentists begin to think about similar cases in their offices and find the confidence necessary to begin referring these patients to you for an evaluation.

Two must-have members in any edentulous study group

To make this group more credible to its members, there are multiple pieces to the puzzle. For starters, as a periodontist or oral surgeon, you will want to include a respected, dental laboratory technician. This person needs to be someone who is not only good at what he or she does but also communicates well, is comfortable in a social setting, and can offer restorative feedback as cases are being discussed from a prosthetic-design prospective. Any good laboratory technician and smart business person will jump at this opportunity right away, as Mr. Bill Grill of Thompson Suburban Dental Laboratory did when Dr. Fred Bye offered him the opportunity. The lab technician will benefit immensely by being the unofficial, de facto laboratory for these cases. There should be no need to pay this person directly for his or her time.

The second key ingredient involves recruiting a doctor who is proficient at full-arch implant restorations. Simply being a prosthodontist does not automatically qualify this person. A prosthodontist with extensive experience in restoring full-arch implant cases has its advantages. But don't rule out the general dentist who has proven experience with restoring full-arch, dental implant-supported prostheses. The key is that this doctor be willing to selflessly impart wisdom to the members of this group without being a snob. This doctor should be humble enough to understand that you, the specialist, are the star of this show.

Perioprosthodontist, Dr. Kevin Murphy of Baltimore, MD, could not play this role better for Dr. Bye. Dr. Murphy is exceptionably skilled in full-arch, implant-supported reconstruction. He is also humble and extremely complimentary of Dr. Bye in the presentations to the group. I completely support the idea of paying this team member a small fee out of respect and so that there is a natural sense of obligation to serve a meaningful purpose. A $2,000 per diem is a reasonable fee.

The edentulous study group's costs and continuing education credits

It is important to keep your costs to a minimum. One of the best ways you can mitigate costs is by holding these meetings at your office. The next, best option would be to hold the meetings at a dental laboratory. You should plan to serve a light, continental breakfast and a decent lunch—usually, something along the lines of Subway or Panera Bread will do. It shouldn't cost you much more than $200 to feed everyone.

Don't spread yourself thin when it comes to your selection of implant companies you will use for these cases. Committing to perform these full-arch procedures with one implant company will give you the ability to leverage that implant company as a partner. In return, ask the same implant company to cover the cost of your implant-restorative expert team member.

If you are not already equipped to offer continuing education (CE) credit, make arrangements with the implant company you will use for these full-arch cases to provide CE credit on your behalf. The local implant representative should be present at each meeting, make sure all doctor names are submitted for CE, and be prepared to address any questions related to the implant system and restorative parts, just as I did for Dr. Bye's group.

The edentulous study group membership tuition

It was usually the doctors who asked me to get them into an implant course for "free" who either skipped out early or failed to show up at all. It may be your natural inclination to offer a free membership to such a group. After all, as long as they refer edentulous patients, you stand to do well on the back end.

In my experience, this is the wrong approach. People place a larger value on what they pay for. If you want your doctors to schedule around these meetings and hold to them, you will do well to create value by charging a reasonable fee, usually in the neighborhood of $500, annually. Most doctors serious about being a part of such a group because of the educational value they'll receive won't mind paying this fee. Unless it is your top referrals who insist on not paying the fee, set the expectation pretty high that each member is expected to pay a nominal fee.

Formal invitation and sales tool

Asking a doctor to pay a fee requires more than a simple e-mail invitation. If you expect doctors to pay for and value your study club, you'll need to present the offer in a formal manner. Hire a professional graphic artist to put the content of your brochure in a professional design. Present the offer professionally, as shown in Figure 5.2, and you will elicit more of a positive response.

The second investment you may choose to make is an investment in each individual group member. The ability to empower each of these doctors with a visual aid is profound. I recommend giving each member a full-arch, dental implant hybrid model as shown in Figure 5.3. These models will cost you about $300 each, but the value they will bring over time in referral loyalty and in full-arch implant patient referrals is unrivaled by most anything else you can give to a referral source. Another advantage that comes with the purchase of multiple models is you can have your practice's name and phone number inscribed on the back of each model.

Duration and frequency of edentulous meetings

For each meeting, you will need enough material to satisfy a 4–6 hour meeting. This is not an evening meeting to be held at the end of a long workday. After seeing patients all day, everyone, including you, is tired and wants to go home to their families and are not prepared in the slightest to think as deeply as you need them to in such a group.

In the Washington, DC, area where I live, most dentists work Monday through Thursday and are off on Friday. Depending on the culture of your region, Friday might be a good day to hold your meetings as well.

Once every 3 months is often enough to hold these meetings, as it gives you plenty of time to build your case presentations in-between each meeting and to make room on your schedule to plan for other professional and direct-to-consumer events that you should be doing also.

The Bye Center Edentulous Patient Implant Prosthetics Study Club

Fred L. Bye, DDS, MS, DABP, DICOI

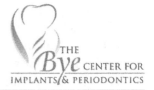

In the U.S. there are more than 30 million adults who are edentulous in at least one arch and this number is expected to grow to 38 million by the year 2020.

As dental professionals we can dramatically change these patients' lives by providing implant supported fixed and removable prostheses. Implant prosthetics enhance edentulous patient's overall health and well-being while restoring their self-image and self-esteem.

Three years ago we formed The Bye Center Edentulous Patient Implant Prosthetics Study Club. During this time, together we have collaborated on the successful rehabilitation of 46 edentulous arches and we will treatment plan 10 new patients during our March Study Club meeting.

In 2014, while continuing to emphasize the surgical and prosthetic treatment options for our edentulous patients, the Study Club will broaden its focus to include partially edentulous implant applications in the esthetic zone.

Dr. Kevin Murphy has agreed to present an organized sequence of lectures relating to implant placement in the esthetic zone. We will include this new sequence of lectures along with our "usual" format of treatment planning cases for full-arch implant prosthetics as well as review completed cases.

We are very fortunate to have Mr. Bill Grill, owner of Thompson Suburban Dental Laboratory, returning to our group. We are also fortunate to welcome another periodontist, Dr. Melanie Chou, to participate with our group.

In order to accommodate our very "full" schedule, our meetings will now start promptly at 7:30am (continental breakfast 7:00am–7:30am) and may not conclude until 3:00pm or 4:00pm.

BioHorizons will co-sponsor our 2014 Study Club Series. For an optimum learning environment the Study Club will remain limited to 20 doctors. For this reason Deena must receive your RSVP to reserve your space by March 10, 2014. 25 CE credit hours total will be issued for the four meetings.

We have an exciting year ahead and I look forward to your participation in the 2014 Edentulous Patient Implant Prosthetics Study Club.

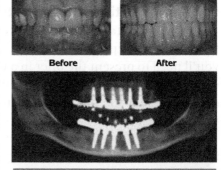

Before   **After**

2014 Study Club Dates:

March 13, 2014	4:00pm–8:00pm
May 2, 2014	7:30am–3:30pm
October 3, 2014	7:30am–3:30pm
December 19, 2014	7:30am–3:30pm

Topics will include:

- Facial Analysis
- Lips and lip movement and their role in gingival-tooth display
- Facial proportions and profiles
- Tooth positions: Midlines, incisal planes, buccal corridors and phonetics
- Treatment of excessive gingival display
- How to establish ideal gingival margin levels
- Biologic width—it's impact with teeth and implants
- Gingival embrasure and papillae management
- Age appropriate vs. white and uncharacterized esthetics
- Pontic form and anterior ridge management
- Single tooth implants and immediate implants
- CAD/Cam all ceramic restorations

Figure 5.2 Example of Dr. Fred Bye's edentulous study group's promotional brochure—by invitation only. Dr. Fred Bye. Reproduced with permission of Dr. Bye.

Fred L. Bye, DDS, MS, DABP, DICOI

Dr. Fred Bye is a leader in the field of implant dentistry. Dr. Bye received his DDS degree and his specialty Masters Degree in Periodonics from the University of Michigan. He was Chief of Periodontics at Shaw AFB Hospital, SC. As a professor at the University of Michigan, Dr. Bye was the Director of Implants for the post graduate periodontal specialty program. Dr. Bye is a board certified Diplomate of the American Board of Periodontology. Dr. Bye is a graduate and Fellow of the Misch Institute, and a Fellow and Diplomate of the International Congress of Oral Implantologists. He is a member of numerous dental implant and periodontal organizations. In 1992, Dr. Bye established the Bye Center for Implants and Periodontics. He is the founder and Director of the Implant Prosthetics for the Edentulous Patient Study Club which focuses on rehabilitating edentulous patients with removable and fixed full arch dental implant prosthetics.

Kevin G. Murphy, DDS, MS

Dr. Kevin Murphy received his dental degree from the University of Illinois where he also received specialty certificates in both Prosthodontics and Periodontics. He also received his master's degree in Oral histology from the same institution. Dr. Murphy is in private practice in Baltimore, Maryland, concentrating in the areas of Prosthodontics, Periodontics and Implant dentistry. He has published numerous articles and textbook chapters on periodontal regeneration and implant dentistry. Dr. Murphy has lectured both nationally and internationally on corticotomy facilitated orthodontia, periodontal and alveolar regeneration, the placement and restoration of dental implants and periodontal prosthesis.

William J. Grill, CDT

William J. Grill, CDT graduated from Loyola College of Maryland in 1975 with a BA in Psychology and a BS in Biology and has earned his CDT in the specialty of implants. His advanced dental studies have been at The Dawson Center for Advancement of Dentistry, the Pankey Institute, and ongoing ASMDT studies at NYU. He is an active member of the International Congress of Oral Implantologists, the American Equilibration Society, and the American Academy of Cosmetic Dentistry. He has spoken for several dental implant companies and numerous study groups. Since 1979, Bill has been the owner/president of Thompson Suburban Dental Lab in Timonium, Maryland, a full service laboratory with an emphasis on implantology and cosmetic dentistry.

PAYMENT INFORMATION
Tuition: $500 (due by March 10, 2014)
Payable to The Bye Center for Implants & Periodontics

VENUE & SCHEDULE
Bye Center for Implants & Periodontics
13424 Pennsylvania Ave., Ste. 201
Hagerstown, MD 21742

March 13, 2014	4:00pm–8:00pm
May 2, 2014	7:30am–3:30pm
October 3, 2014	7:30am–3:30pm
December 19, 2014	7:30am–3:30pm

RSVP by March 10, 2014
By invitation only
Contact Deena Anderson
13424 Pennsylvania Ave., Ste. 201
Hagerstown, MD 21742
tel: 866.739.6868
fax: 301.790.4990
deena@periodonticsandimplants.com

Cosponsored by

BIOHORIZONS®

Academy of General Dentistry
25 CE Credits

PACE
Program Approved for Continuing Education

Name: _____

Address: _____

City / State / Zip: _____

Phone: (_____) _____ Fax: (_____) _____

Payment Method:
Check (enclosed payable to The Bye Center for Implants & Periodontics) ☐   Credit Card ☐

Total amount enclosed: $ _____

☐ Visa   ☐ MC   ☐ Discover   #: _____

Expiration Date: _____ / _____ / _____   CVV ____ ____ ____ ____

Cardholder Name: _____

Billing Address: _____

Approved PACE Program Provider FAGD/MAGD Credit Approval does not imply acceptance by a state or provincial board of dentistry or AGD endorsement. The current term of approval extends from 6/1/2013-5/31/2016. Provider #219038

SPMP14006 REV A FEB 2014

Figure 5.2 (*Continued*)

If you believe you have the capacity to run an edentulous study group, I encourage you to begin putting such a group together—immediately. Everyone involved will benefit enormously, none more than the increased number of edentulous patients you will treat.

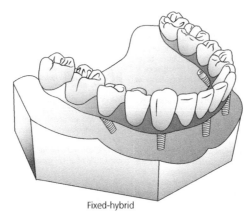

Fixed-hybrid

Figure 5.3 Providing each member with such a model will help them sell cases.

Target your top two to five referral sources' patient base

Now, let's get into another strategy that will undoubtedly attract more patients from your referral sources. Think of all the referring dentists you work with. Now, think of those few who refer you the most dental implant patients. What percentage of your overall referral base do they represent? I'd be willing to bet it's less than 20%. This is the Pareto principle, also known as the "80–20 rule," which states that 80% of the results come from just 20% of the effort or resources.

Your best implant referral sources are within the smaller 20% group. They reside within this smaller group for at least two primary reasons: (i) These referring doctors believe in implant dentistry to the fullest. (ii) They also believe that you are the best choice for their patients when it comes to implant surgery and bedside manners and so on. In a nutshell, the fact is that these doctors place a great deal of trust and faith in you.

Focus on your top 20% referral sources

Your top 20% referral source is exactly the type of referral source you will want to target for more dental implant patients. Believe it or not, there are still literally hundreds of patients with missing teeth in their practices who are still unaware of dental implants and the benefits dental implants will bring to the quality of their lives. Part of

Box 5.2 Such a letter is out to your top referral sources' patients on your top referral sources' letterhead.

Best general dental office ever letterhead

Dear Mrs. [patient last name],

Did you know that missing teeth not only affects your smile but also leads to the loss of bone in the lower one-third of your face? Missing teeth might also negatively influence you to avoid certain nutrient-rich foods, since you may be unable to chew properly.

Replacing missing teeth with dental implants has become one of the most requested procedures in my practice. Dental implant patients regain their ability to properly chew their food; project a healthy, confident smile; and stop the rapid bone loss that missing teeth can cause.

In association with Dr. Implant Surgeon, a respected local [periodontist or oral surgeon], we are making available to you a free dental implant consultation and examination. Once [Dr. Periodontist or Oral Surgeon] and I have gathered the required information, we will present you with a treatment plan that will detail your options.

To take advantage of this complementary evaluation, contact [Dr. Periodontist or Oral Surgeon's] office at (777) 777-7777 to schedule an appointment today. I have also enclosed a referral form for his office. Let his/her staff know I referred you for the dental implant consultation, and his $250 examination fee will be waived through [expiration date].

As always, thank you for choosing Superior Dental Care. I look forward to seeing you soon.

Sincerely,
Dr. General Dentist

---

your job is to help your top referral sources make their patients more aware of the benefits of dental implants.

The process works like magic when done right and kept simple. By simple, I mean sending out a letter to the dentist's patient base. Box 5.2 is an example of how such a letter might flow. You can word this letter as you see fit, but such a letter only works like a charm if patients think that it's coming from their dentists, not you, the specialist. This letter should be personalized on your referral sources' letterhead, not yours.

You might ask, "My best referrals are already doing well, so why not use this with the dentists who aren't such good referral sources and make them better?" This is a great question. Your "so-so" referrals are so-so for multiple reasons, which I won't get into here. But this effort won't make an average-referring dentist any better, and in most cases, an average-referring dentist won't appreciate these efforts, anyway. The 80–20 rule is designed around putting 80% of your efforts behind that 20% who are responsible for 80% of your good results. Therefore, the focus must remain with your top 20% referral base, not the 80% who are only responsible for 20% of your implant business. Makes sense?

Take responsibility for all associated costs and logistics

This is meant to be your idea and your request. For this reason, it is important that you take complete responsibility for managing this process in every way. For this to work, you have to be in control of planting the seed, watering the seed, and harvesting the crop.

This means you will pay for the printing of the letter on your referrals' letterhead, the stuffing of the envelopes, and the postage for mailing the letter. Remember, this is not one of your typical referrals. This is a top 20% referral source that plays a meaningful role in producing 80% of your overall implant business. No amount of money spent on this project can match the value that your top referring dentists already bring.

As much as you understand the benefit to your own practice, your referring doctor should feel like you are investing in his or her practice as well, because essentially you are. When patients begin showing up for their appointments and asking your referring dentist more questions about replacing missing teeth with dental implants, the referring dentist will no doubt realize the value you bring to his or her office as a specialist.

Patients and professionals are used to direct to consumer advertising

"Everyone knows dental professional specialists don't market directly to the patient" is the response I received from an oral surgeon I encouraged to go direct to consumer. From a traditional sense, he was right. The question is, are you willing to break with tradition if it means benefiting more patients and performing more implant surgical procedures than you will if you continue to solely rely on professional referrals?

In this modern marketing world, it is totally acceptable for virtually any traditional business to business to advertise and promote directly to the consumer. When I grew up in the 1970s and 1980s, it was rare to see a pharmaceutical company advertise their prescription drugs on television. Physicians relied on the pharmaceutical rep to detail the drugs far more than they do today. Chances were very good that the patient never heard of the drug until the physician wrote the prescription.

Today, in the 2000s, no one does direct to consumer marketing more than pharmaceutical companies. Long before the physician writes a prescription, the patient might have already self-diagnosed based on symptoms presented in the TV advertisements. So now, patients are requesting prescriptions for specific medications they have never used before. I can hardly enjoy a Sunday afternoon pro football game without exposing my curious 11-year-old son to commercials for all types of ailments and dysfunctions. I keep waiting for him to ask me something like, "Dad, what's the difference between Viagra® and Cialis®?"

You've probably seen the orthopedic companies such as Smith & Nephew® advertising their hip-replacement devices or BIOMET® advertising their partial knee-replacement implants by going direct to consumer through television ads. How are they successful in these efforts? After all, it's not like the consumer in need can pick up a loaf of bread and a new knee replacement down at the local supermarket! But this type of advertising works in their favor in at least two ways. Their ads build credibility, for the company, with prospective doctors who are capable of prescribing and using these products on their patients. Additionally, the general public's inquires about these products during their medical appointments can go a long way as well.

You too should go direct to consumer

I've never been in favor of the specialty practice that makes a conscious choice to rely 100% on the local general dental community for their dental implant patients. Trust me, I get it; there are certain procedures you will forever remain dependent on professional referral sources for, just as you should. But implant dentistry is a different animal than procedures such as *third-molar extractions* or *esthetic-crown lengthening.* Does the patient who can't tolerate their partial really need a general dentist to tell them they might be a candidate for dental implants? Of course not.

Those patients can come directly to you, the specialist, and you can tell them if they are candidates for implants any day of the week. You can then turn around and work with their dentists (if they have one) or work with your restorative doctor of choice to complete the case. Anything less than this approach makes you, as a specialist, too dependent on professional relationships that quite frankly can be enormously volatile based on personality clashes, misunderstandings, and too many other superficial variables that can affect a dentist's decision to refer a patient or not.

Professional referrals should serve as just one way you go about attracting new implant patients to your practice. No top referring dentist will be disappointed when you suddenly have the ability to refer out as much implant-restorative business as you take in implant surgery. Everyone wins when you begin to attract implant patients directly.

Strategies for going direct to consumer

Now, you ask, "How do I bypass the dentist and promote my specialty practice direct to patient?" My recommendation is that you begin offering patient education seminars immediately.

Patient education seminars are a powerful tool for specialists

I feel so strongly about this marketing concept that I dedicated a whole chapter to it and therefore won't cover any details here. But if you have not already read Chapter 2 as a specialist in particular, I encourage you to do so and begin hosting these seminars in your office immediately.

In the spirit of going direct to consumer, consider the power that a well-oiled, patient education seminar will give you. Having a patient education seminar will allow you, as a specialist, to advertise your implant business on the radio, in the newspaper, and by partnering up with your local GP offices in ways that you may find otherwise diffi-cult to do. With patient education seminars, you have the best of both worlds. You can advertise on the radio to the general public, and

Box 5.3 A letter should be sent to most area restorative dentists explaining your plans to host patient education seminars.

Dear Dr. General Dentist [personalize],

While dental implants continue to become a more accepted teeth replacement modality by the general public, there are still only about 5% of all prospective patients being treated with dental implants. Some of this has to do with finances, but much of it has to do with the fact that most people are simply unaware of this option.

I believe the greater part of the responsibility remains with us as oral healthcare providers to educate the general public on the ill effects of missing teeth and the long-term solutions that dental implants can provide to many of these individuals.

Over the coming 12-month period, I have decided to offer free patient education seminars on the subject of dental implants in my office once per month. This seminar is designed to be patient friendly and will address the following topics:

- Why missing teeth lead to bone loss
- How dental implants help to stop excessive bone loss caused by missing teeth
- Before-and-after images of dental implant restorations
- Examples of implant-supported fixed and removable overdentures
- General processes required for receiving dental implants
- Costs associated with dental implants

We encourage you to invite your patients to attend our next seminar on November 6, 2014, by providing them with the enclosed passes. We do not perform restorative procedures in our practice and will be sure to sing your praises when we know a patient is attending from your office. Each attendee will be given dental implant education materials to take home and review. We will encourage each patient to consult with his or her dentist for restorative advice on moving forward with implants.

Thank you in advance for your interest in our patient education seminars.

Signed,
You [personalize]

you can target your area restorative dentists and encourage them to recommend your seminars to their patients.

For example, it can be very powerful to send out a letter such as in Box 5.3 to your local general dental community once per month. If done right, once these patients attend your seminar, the odds rise dramatically that they will choose you to perform their dental implant surgery. Send these patients back to their restorative doctors for the implant restorations and watch your professional relationships soar with such dentists.

Using an ad agency for your advertising

Early on in this process, I suggested you go through a reputable advertising agency. This way, the ad agency can do all the background research for you and come up with the radio station(s) that best fit the demographic you are targeting and the bottom-line fees. A good ad agency understands that it is in their best interest to maintain a lasting relationship with you and therefore desires to work on your behalf to achieve the best results with your advertising dollars.

Leverage the advertising agency; they are the experts when it comes to picking radio stations, newspapers, and magazines, depending on what you are advertising. If a radio or print ad isn't generating enough new business for you, that ad agency should work on your behalf to either renegotiate the advertising fees or recommend eliminating the ad altogether and perhaps doing a new one.

Track every method of advertising you produce so that you can compare what you spend on your specific ads with what your ads generate in implant treatment. The best way to track the value of your advertisements is through your patient database software, as discussed in Chapter 6.

The prosthodontist specialty

If you are a prosthodontist and you perform advanced, dental implant surgery for a general dentist referral base, each of the afore-mentioned strategies are most certainly applicable to you also. On the flip side, if you are a prosthodontist focusing on the more advanced implant restorations (not surgery), it is worth it to outline some approaches you can take as a specialist that are unique to your advanced, restorative skill set.

Assuming you are not a threat to other specialists for implant surgery, you can set yourself up to become the go-to restorative clinician for many of the nonreferral cases that randomly end up in oral surgeons' and periodontists' offices. The dental community already regards you as the restorative authority. Even certain members of the general dental community that understand their restorative limitations will begin to refer their more challenging implant cases to you when you begin to apply these marketing strategies as a restorative specialist.

Process of reciprocation

As a prosthodontist, there are several strategies you can implement to target oral surgeons and periodontists. Perhaps the greatest leverage you have is your ability to spread the wealth of patient referrals among a few choice oral surgeons and periodontists who you prefer to work with. Your goal should be to routinely refer out the implant surgeries to these specialists. The law of reciprocity will dictate that the more implant surgeries you refer out, the more implant restorations you will receive from this core group of surgical specialists.

To best position yourself for this, you will need to be acquiring new, prospective, dental implant patients directly through your direct to consumer marketing efforts on a regular basis. This means you will need a very effective direct to patient strategy for attracting them. If you follow the guidelines I have outlined in this book, it will not be an issue for you to maintain a constant stream of new dental implant patients.

Prosthetically driven implant white papers

The other thing I would recommend any restorative-driven prosthodontist do is to write white papers. The more ways you can separate yourself clinically, and document it in the process, the more you become the expert on that subject. And one of the best and simplest ways you can document your fine work is by writing white papers.

Don't wait for some well-known dental publication to publish your article. Write a white paper and distribute the article yourself. If you need to understand the proper guidelines of writing a white paper, go to www.klariti.com. For about $10.00, they will give you the guidelines on writing a white paper in multiple formats.

A white paper can help build credibility and demonstrate an implant clinician's skill set in a way that is professional and respected by your restorative and surgical colleagues. The subject of your white paper should be compelling to its audience and advanced in nature. Don't waste your time doing a white paper on, say, a simple, two-unit, posterior implant case.

Two procedures that would benefit you to write white papers on are full-arch, immediate- (or delayed-) occlusal loading and dental implant restorations in the esthetic zone. Look for different angles with each case. One case might be a hybrid prosthesis with a titanium base and acrylic teeth, while another might be a full-arch, zirconia bridge as the final prosthesis to an immediate-occlusal load case you performed with your surgical specialist of choice. You might have performed two e.max® crowns on two maxillary central incisor implants that turned out beautifully. Document it with great images and do a white paper on it.

When done right, white papers are not perceived as a sales pitch because they are designed to educate and help your readers solve problems. In the process of educating your prospective referral sources (i.e., surgical specialists), as the clinician behind the white paper, you gain favor—you become the expert. As more of these cases find their way to oral surgeons' and periodontists' practices—independent of their referral sources—you become the go-to clinician for the restorative phase, guaranteed to work like a charm.

Role of an implant coordinator

I have worked with some very good implant coordinators. Some are particularly skilled and knowledgeable at implant surgical and restorative protocols across multiple systems, while others are exceptional at manipulating CBCT surgical images and designing treatment plan presentations and administrating public relations. But generally speaking, most specialists don't maximize the implant coordinator position to its full potential.

World-class speakers like Dr. Mark Setter, a periodontist; JoAn Majors, author of *Open the Door – To Your Purpose in Implant Dentistry*; and Kathi Carlson, co-creator of *The Implant Consortium*, are far and away among those individuals I respect most when it comes to understanding the makeup of a proficient implant coordinator. And while my level of understanding on what it takes to develop a true implant coordinator will never rival the practical experiences of the aforementioned respected dental professionals, I would venture to say my appreciation for this role will rival most anyone. Box 5.4 includes some important roles an implant coordinator should be able to perform.

Box 5.4 Some key roles an implant coordinator should play.

Implant coordinator

- Coordinates clinical communications between the implant surgical office and referring/restorative dentists, including date of implant placement, number of implants placed, restorative platform sizes, estimated date of integration, date implants are ready for restoration, delivery of impression copings, and laboratory analogs (to referring dentists)
- Coordinates all aspects of implant-related internal marketing including assuring the front desk staff has the appropriate verbal skills, making available patient education materials (implant brochures, implant models/typodonts, implant flip charts, etc.), and administering implant animations to patients
- Coordinates all aspects of implant marketing and education to dental professionals, including staff lunch-and-learn presentations, implant study groups, and prospecting for new patient referral sources
- Processes CBCT raw data and begins initial virtual positioning of implants (to be finalized by surgeon)
- Coordinates direct to consumer marketing

You can hire an implant coordinator outright or if you have the right person in your office, you might place that staff member in this position. If you choose the latter, initially gain agreement from this staff member to take on some expanded "implant" duties while maintaining the current role as a dental assistant, or front desk receptionist, or office manager, and so on. As this staff member begins to develop a flow and shows signs of success, you can then look to replace his or her current position and promote this person to the full-time implant coordinator position. For the right person, in the right specialty practice, this is easily a full-time position. However you choose to get there and depending on how much you would like to grow your implant business, this position is a wise investment if you intend to implement much of what you have learned in this chapter.

Characteristics of a proficient implant coordinator include someone that is organized, manages multiple tasks well, has a pleasing personality, is smart enough to understand surgical and restorative protocols in implant dentistry, and is articulate, expressive, and driven for success.

From the delivery of restorative parts to the management of the direct to consumer education seminars schedule, your implant coordinator must play a big part in the success of your implant business. Hiring the right person for this position requires that this individual be compensated well. To keep this person driven will usually require sharing in the success and goals of the implant practice. Similar to an implant sales representative who usually has a base salary plus commissions, I like the idea of giving this individual a salary and an incentive based on the office reaching certain realistic implant goals.

Don't make the mistake of setting goals that are unattainable because you tried to grow your numbers too big, too fast. That said, set goals that will make you and your implant coordinator stretch together. For instance, if for the past 12-month period you've averaged 75 implants placed per quarter, or 300 implants for the year, once you have in place much of what is advised in this chapter, your goal for the next quarter might be to grow by only ten implants to a total of 85 implants for the quarter. Once this goal is met, the second quarter's goal might be to grow by an additional 15 implants to 100 implants total for the quarter. In your third quarter, you may add another 30 implants on top of your second quarter's total.

By the time you approach the fourth quarter, with the established momentum, you will find it very realistic to grow your business by another 45 implants for the quarter. Now, you and your implant coordinator have reached your goal of growing your implant business by 100 implants to a total number of 400 implants over the past 12-month period.

Expand your geographical range

Why box yourself into a small corner when you are capable of so much more? There is no good reason a particularly skilled oral surgeon in Tampa, FL, can't attract certain implant patients from as far as 375 miles away in Panama City, FL, or a periodontist in Houston, TX, can't attract patients from as far as 260 miles away in Kerrville, TX.

I didn't say you should routinely expect patients from distant referral sources, but if you have exceptional specialized clinical skills, not possessed by the average surgical specialist, you can position yourself in the marketplace to pull implant referrals from a much larger geographic pool than your immediate competitors. At the advice of their dentist (or physician—see Chapter 3), many patients will travel from one end of the state to another or even across the country if the case is challenging enough and it means receiving the very best of care. You have to first carve your niche and become a noted expert.

It starts with good documentation of your advanced bone/ soft tissue-grafting and implant cases. For instance, a hip graft on a severely atrophic mandible that others might write off as being hopeless can now be restored beautifully on five implants because of your noted reliability in such cases or a maxillary case that has sustained blunt force trauma and wiped out the central and lateral incisors on a supermodel-type, gorgeous 25-year-old female. Largely because of your ability to reestablish the foundation and work with choice restorative clinicians and master ceramists, it is possible to restore such a patient's natural beauty and smile.

These are the types of cases that will find you from great distances, but you must document and write case reports and white papers. Hire ghostwriters if you must, but get these reports into the hands of every dentist within your state and neighboring state(s). Repurpose your case reports into a blog that you send out to your growing e-mail list of dentists. Share these same cases in dental groups on the professional social media network, LinkedIn, and dialogue with doctors who ask questions and make comments. Submit these case reports for publication. It's never been easier to make your expertise known to the masses. Do so and you will draw patients from near and far.

Reducing clinical limitations is crucial

As a nonclinician, I may not be qualified to advise you on the ins and outs of performing any particular procedure, but here is what I can tell you. Today, you compete against the specialist and the general practitioner for implant surgery. The best tool any specialist can incorporate to support his or her marketing efforts, in this increasingly competitive market, is an advanced surgical skill set. Being capable of performing the more difficult implant surgical procedures is a must. Let's consider some of the more advanced procedures most surgical specialists should be capable of performing.

Immediate anterior provisional

In the anterior region, there is a limited opportunity to manage the soft tissue and maintain a natural scallop and papilla around a dental implant crown. Using a healing abutment on, say, an implant placed in the central incisor position is no longer considered your best option for achieving this goal, so as a rule, stop doing it. I have heard countless renowned implant surgeons echo this fact in the literature and from the podium. One of my surgical specialists who has made this concept a marketing staple in his Crofton, MD, practice is Dr. David Mugford, a periodontist. Renowned clinicians like periodontists Dr. Paul Fugazzotto and Dr. Maurice Salama have lectured on this in their respective courses for years. Immediate provisionals in the anterior region can separate you from your competition.

Immediate-occlusal loading

Full-arch, immediate-occlusal loading is highly successful and is here to stay. Dr. Peter Moy, Dr. Paulo Malo, Dr. Hamid Shafie, and other renowned figures lecture on this subject around the world. Surgeons who do the best job of making their experience in these procedures known to the local dental community will continue to attract the growing number of restorative doctors that influence their patients to opt for a fixed, full-arch implant prosthesis on the same day as the surgery. If you are still careful not to advocate this procedure because you fear the implants will fail or you have not been adequately trained in it, you will lose implant business for sure. Implant success rates for this procedure are consistent with traditional implant placement, 97%. I encourage you to seek out a credible course and become confident in this procedure.

Bone regeneration

When you have world-class, bone-grafting experts and teachers like Dr. Michael Pikos, Dr. John Russo, Dr. Craig Misch, Dr. Daniel Spagnoli, and so on willing to offer you priceless techniques and the wisdom it took years to achieve, there is really no good reason for not being able to grow bone for the proper dental implant size and positioning. To market your specialty implant business effectively requires that you be capable of regenerating significant vertical bone loss, significant buccal wall defects, severely pneumatized sinuses, and so on because these are all complications with successful surgical solutions. There are countless case reports and multiple courses offered on the subject of advanced bone grafting. Whether it is using ridge-splitting techniques, harvesting autogenous bone, or incorporating SonicWeld™ with allograft bone materials or plasma-rich growth factors (PRGF®) or even using rhBMP-2 (Infuse®), when faced with certain challenges, your ability to regenerate the required bone is what is expected of you as a specialist.

Soft tissue regeneration

It doesn't matter if you are a periodontist, a prosthodontist, or an oral surgeon, if you are performing implant surgery anywhere near the esthetic zone, to be competitive, you need to have a thorough understanding of how to best manage soft tissue around dental implants. One of the foremost soft tissue-grafting textbooks, *Soft Tissue and Esthetic Considerations in Implant Therapy*, was not written by a periodontist; it was written by Dr. Anthony Sclar, an oral surgeon. Who says you have to be a periodontist to master soft tissue concepts around implants? Maybe it was the same person who said you have to be an oral surgeon to perform advanced, bone-grafting procedures. If you are an oral surgeon, it behooves you to become as much the go-to surgeon for the missing central incisor as your competing periodontists. Today, you are less likely to receive a referral because you are capable of placing implants and more likely to receive a referral because the dentist can bank on what the soft tissue will look like around your implants once the case is complete.

Complications in implant dentistry

Any general dentist routinely restoring dental implants has had dental implant problems—guaranteed. As a specialist, you will do well by your practice to be recognized as the doctor capable of surgically fixing dental implant-related problems. Many of these implants can be repaired successfully—for a fee; others will need to be replaced. Position yourself as an authority in implant complications, and you will profit from these cases either way.

Periodontist Dr. Paul Petrungaro penned a great case report on peri-implantitis in the May 2013 issue of *Inside Dentistry*; Dr. Carl Misch lectures on *Implant Complications* around the world; and a great book on the subject is titled, *Dental Implant Complications: Etiology, Prevention and Treatment*, written by Dr. Stuart J. Froum, with a host of contributors.

Fully guided surgery

Undoubtedly, you have heard the best and the brightest say from the podium that "implant dentistry is a restorative discipline with a surgical component." With guided surgery, you have the ability to truly plan your cases and position your implants from a restorative-driven perspective. Guided surgery allows you to think the case through once and then freeze your plan in place by ordering a computer-generated guide to manifest your plan. If you currently plan your implant cases with the use of a CBCT image, guided surgery won't require any more planning time, but it will significantly cut your surgical chair time and simultaneously improve your placement accuracy. Imagine placing four adjacent implants in a free-end, posterior mandibular edentulous site and having the implants properly spaced mesial distally and optimally positioned buccal–lingual for the best possible axial load and restoration, all in about 15–20 minutes, each and every time. Dr. Scott Ganz, editor in chief of *Cone Beam International Magazine of Cone Beam Dentistry*, is one of the most brilliant minds that I have witnessed lecture on the subject. Aside from the fact that guided surgery will make you a more restorative-driven surgeon, this technique will also bring marketing value to your practice. A good reference guide on the subject is *The Art of Computer-Guided Implantology* by Drs. Philippe B. Tardieu and Alan L. Rosenfeld.

Summary

Change is inevitable; change has its own price, and to a greater extent, the price of complacency is far more expensive than change itself. The sooner you act on this fact, the sooner you position your specialty implant business for major growth.

There is no good reason any specialist should be unsettled by the number of general dentists choosing to perform dental implant surgery. The dental implant market as a whole remains very much untapped, and there will always be an abundance of available treatment to go around for everyone. There are multiple avenues any specialist, with a solid clinical skill set, can take to achieve exponential growth in implant dentistry. Traditional approaches for cultivating professional relationships, like study groups, produce superior professional referral results when such groups are designed to generate meaningful involvement from its membership, as with Dr. Fred Bye's edentulous study group. Surgical specialists will also do very well to incorporate nontraditional marketing efforts, such as going direct to consumer, by hosting dental implant seminars.

You only compete with other specialists and general dentists for implant business when you choose to limit your marketing effort to the same mediocre strategies that your specialist counterparts choose.

CHAPTER 6

Database marketing

In an era where most every practitioner places great emphasis on gaining more and more new patients, one of the most difficult challenges I face in coaching implant marketing clients is having doctors understand exactly how valuable their patient databases are. Instead of making a concerted effort to target their patient databases for dental implants, they would rather place untold resources behind looking for new patients, cutting supplies costs, looking for countless ways to help patients use their $1,000 dental insurance maximum, and so on.

No one will argue against the value of a steady stream of new patients or keeping costs down, but why not channel equal effort on the very things that will position you to perform more dental implant procedures? I've always said that since rapport and trust must first be established with every new patient, the most willing dental implant prospective patient is the patient of record who still needs treatment. You have trust with your current patients. Since they still need more of your services, why not mine your patients of record like a prospector mines for gold? If you do so, you will perform far more dental implants than you ever thought were possible.

Take a lesson from Blockbuster® Video's founder, David P. Cook, who had already made his fortune in the petroleum industry in great part through his ability to manage large databases. Blockbuster has since gone out of business, but at the height of its success in 2004

Marketing Implant Dentistry: Attract and Influence Patients to Accept Your Dental Implant Treatment Plan, First Edition. Marcus Hines.
© 2016 John Wiley & Sons, Inc. Published 2016 by John Wiley & Sons, Inc.

when they had more than 60,000 employees and over 9,000 stores worldwide, within their niche they were unstoppable. From the beginning, Cook understood that if he applied many of the same database principles to movie rentals, there was no reason he couldn't take the movie rental business by storm. In the fall of 1985 when Cook opened his first location, the store was mobbed with eager customers wanting to do business.

Cook was masterful at targeting specific demographics and piquing their unique cinematic interests. He knew that when he opened a store in inner-city Detroit, Michigan, the "new release" section, display signs, and inventory of select movie titles had better represent that demographic's interests, which would be different from the Blockbuster location in suburbia Potomac, Maryland. His data systems were so tight that based on the median age, socioeconomic status, ethnicity, and other factors, he could have a new store opened and appropriately stocked for that specific demographic in 24 hours (Graslie, 2013).

Successful marketers like David Cook understand the power of serving demographics on a much deeper level than the average business owner. Database marketing at its best is like shooting fish in a barrel. The same database marketing principles Cook used to make millions in the petroleum industry are the same principles he used to revolutionize the way movies were rented on a massive scale. These principles are universal. In relative terms, if Cook was passionate about implant dentistry and were to apply the same principles of database marketing to the business of implant dentistry, he would be equally successful.

The more you know about a collective group, the better you are positioned to tailor your marketing efforts so that your message resonates with that group. And the more your message resonates, the bigger the catch you will make with the least amount of effort.

In your case, the more your patients trust you have their best interests at heart, the more they will find a way to say "yes" to your sincere implant recommendations. This formula is simple, scientific, and totally applicable to dental implant case acceptance.

This is why it is important to have systems in place that prevent you from being emotional about dental implant treatment plans for your patients. If you have comprehensive data about your patients with missing teeth and a strategy for consistently communicating the benefits of implant dentistry to the same patients, you cannot lose.

Automate your data entry as much as possible

Your database has the potential to be golden, but if you are like most doctors, you don't feed your database pertinent details about every patient's visit. It is these details that will allow you to target market your patients with missing teeth so well that you will be surprised by the growing number of patients who tell you they are ready for dental implants. Arriving at this point requires at least two key components with the first being good quality practice management software.

In a January 2014 article titled "Choosing the right dental practice management software," Dr. Claudio M. Levato said, "There are many [practice management] solutions from which to choose that will deliver excellent results; the quality of the results achieved will depend upon how well the user implements the program's resources and solutions" (Levato, 2014). Dr. Levato went on to say that "The vast majority of dentists still only use a fraction of the applications they have already purchased." This leads me to the second key component, which is data entry. This means having a constant feeding of factual details into your software, one patient and one appointment at a time.

You need to know how many teeth your patients are missing on average. You need to know which teeth your patients are missing the most. You need to know how long your patients have been missing their teeth or what type of prostheses your patients are wearing. You need to know what percentage of your patients have replaced their missing teeth or not and how many of your patients are wearing a partial denture, a full-denture plate, or both. You need to know how long it's been since each of your endodontically treated patients received a root canal, post and core, and/or crown, compared to the average life span of the endodontically treated tooth.

When you make a concerted effort to input all facets of treatment through your practice management software, you suddenly have the ability to spit out pertinent data in a report for the purposes of creating a target marketing campaign. This will set you on a whole new trajectory when it comes to case acceptance. No one has helped me to understand this more than Ms. DeVon Banks, owner of the consulting firm D-TECH Business Concepts, LLC, and authority on data entry/ management.

DeVon says, "When you chart your patients, chart them through your practice management software. When you create treatment plans, enter the data for your treatment plans into your practice management software. And when you perform a treatment walkout, don't bypass the standard protocols put in place by your practice management software for the sake of convenience. Perform your walkouts through your practice management software by extracting the procedures you performed from the original treatment plan that you entered into the system."

DeVon's message is profound. In other words, if your treatment plan was for a socket graft and dental implant, by walking out the patient's treatment through the treatment plan, you automatically update your invaluable database. This allows you to run accurate reports on how many socket grafts and dental implant surgical procedures you have treatment planned for, how many you have actually performed, and which of your patients still require these procedures.

If you can't retrieve such invaluable information for the purposes of evaluating your dental implant potential, you're probably suffering from "garbage in, garbage out." Establish systems that naturally allow for the accumulation of vital information about every patient visit on a daily basis, and over time, this accumulated data will empower you beyond belief.

Querying your removable partial-denture patients for in-depth insight

Obviously, there are multiple categories of patients who have missing teeth that you will want to examine in your practice. I cannot possibly begin to explore each of these categories in detail here. I will give you a thorough example that you can apply to most categories of missing teeth and immediately begin working with patients already in your practice.

Let's examine a hypothetical database of patients who were treated with a removable partial-denture (RPD) for demonstration purposes only. When I say hypothetically, I'm only talking about these specific statistics, but know that the realities of such statistics are very real. Such a query can be made as detailed and complex as necessary to extract the information you need to know, but for the purposes of this exercise (and in an effort to keep your interest), here, we will keep it as simple as possible.

Box 6.1 There is an abundance of missing teeth in this category.

RPD patient database query

- Number of patients wearing an RPD = 223
- Number of male versus female patients = 99 males and 124 females
- Median age = 55
- Average number of years patient has worn current RPD = 5.2
- Average number of missing teeth = 5.6
- Average number of years patient in RPD group has been a patient of record = 6.2
- Birthdates/Anniversary (more on use of birthdates/anniversaries later in this chapter)

Since we have chosen to query all RPD patients as our missing-teeth category (Box 6.1), we now need to understand the data. When we analyze the results of this query, for starters, we discover there are 223 RPD patients with an average of 5.6 missing teeth. This means that within this very small, segmented portion of the practice, there are 1249 missing teeth. Did you hear me? One thousand two-hundred and forty-nine missing teeth between only 223 of this practice's patients is what I just said! Remember this 1249 number as I will make references to it later in the chapter.

Our query also reveals that the median age of this RPD group is 55 years old. This represents a relatively young age group since today the probability that this group will live well into their 80s and 90s is very good since a non-smoker, on average, can expect to reach the age of 85.

Most of the RPD patients in this query are females, which means, on average, most of these patients can expect to live at least another 26 years. What are the chances their RPD will last another 26 years beyond the 5.2 years that they have already worn it? The literature certainly doesn't support it. Since the average RPD patient in this query has already had their removable prosthesis for more than 5 years, it is very reasonable to believe a significant percentage of these patients' RPDs are no longer functioning properly.

Now that we know which patients in this practice's database fit the category of wearing an RPD, we are much closer to designing a marketing campaign to target this group for dental implants on a monthly basis. That said, we're not quite there just yet. While we understand the numbers (1249 edentulous sites), it is equally important that we get a feel for what the patients' experiences with their RPDs have been. Once we have a deeper sense of how patients feel about their RPDs, we can then tailor our marketing message accordingly.

Collecting the right data through patient surveys is crucial

If the aforementioned *queries* suggest there is a market for what we desire to help more patients with (in this case, implant dentistry), then *surveying* the patients will tell us how we should best package our marketing efforts to promote the service we intend to provide.

The doctor has the ability to know everything about their patients' oral health so that they can best influence their patients to accept their treatment plans. This is any marketer's dream! The more you know about a person, the greater the chances you will seal the deal and influence that person to make a wise decision.

Consider President Barack Obama's campaign for reelection in 2012. His campaign data collection was executed masterfully and ended up playing a major role in his team's ability to raise $1.06 billion and ultimately bring about his reelection.

The campaign manager, Jim Messina, said, "We are going to measure every single thing in this campaign." The data accumulated through surveys was so telling that it helped their fund-raising committees design contests around facts like West Coast females between the ages of 40 and 49 would make significantly higher campaign contributions if it meant possibly winning a dinner with both George Clooney and President Obama. No hunch is going to help you arrive at this conclusion!

There is no excuse for ignoring how your patients of record feel about their teeth replacement prostheses as a collective group. The only way you will truly know how your patients feel about this area of their oral health is to ask them in the form of a survey as demonstrated in Box 6.2. The results of the respondents should be documented.

Box 6.2 Each category of missing-teeth patients should be surveyed separately. This questionnaire happens to be for RPD patients.

RPD patient questionnaire

1 What is your age?
   ○ 18–24   ○ 35–44   ○ 55–64   ○ 75 or older
   ○ 25–34   ○ 45–54   ○ 65–74

2 Approximately how long have you worn a removable partial denture?
   ○ Less than 1 year   ○ 8–10 years
   ○ 1–4 years   ○ 11–15 years
   ○ 5–7 years   ○ 16 or more years

3 How do you feel about your removable partial denture?
   ○ I am quite pleased with my removable partial denture.
   ○ I am somewhat pleased with my removable partial denture.
   ○ I don't really care for my removable partial denture, but I tolerate it.
   ○ I don't care for my removable partial denture at all and rarely wear it, if ever.

4 Please tell us which of the following problems you are experiencing, if any, associated with your removable partial denture (please select as many answers that apply to you):
   ○ My removable partial denture moves when I chew my food.
   ○ I am embarrassed to remove my removable partial denture at night.
   ○ I don't particularly care for the way my removable partial denture looks.
   ○ Food gets trapped beneath my removable partial denture.
   ○ I am not experiencing problems associated with my removable partial denture.
   ○ Others (please specify)

   [   ]

5 Please tell us what you like about your removable partial denture (select as many answers that apply to you):
   ○ My removable partial denture helps me to chew my food better.
   ○ My removable partial denture improves my smile.
   ○ My removable partial denture feels very natural.
   ○ There is nothing I really like about my removable partial denture.
   ○ Others (please specify)

   [   ]

6 What is the life span of a partial denture that you would consider to be acceptable?
   ○ Less than 5 years   ○ Between 16 and 20 years
   ○ Between 5 and 10 years   ○ 20 years or more
   ○ Between 11 and 15 years

7 Do you generally wear your removable partial denture to bed at night?
  ○ Yes   ○ No

8 Do you use some form of denture adhesive (Poligrip, Fixodent, etc.) with your removable partial denture?
  ○ Yes   ○ No
  If Yes, which brand or product do you use?

How you structure your survey is important

Designing survey questions is a skill set, but it's a skill that can be acquired. Like anything else, the more you do, the better you become at it. One of the most basic guidelines about surveying is the importance of refraining from any bias in your questions. In other words, don't try to lead the person you are questioning down a path to give you the answers you are looking for—that's not research. Just because you succeeded in getting those you surveyed to give you the answers you were looking for, doesn't mean you have the answers you need to best structure your marketing plan.

If most of your patients are happy with their RPDs because they function well and look great, your survey should be capable of revealing this to you, too, regardless of your desire to perform more dental implant procedures. Incidentally, such answers would not eliminate these patients as ideal candidates for dental implants, since we know dental implants are the best alternative for teeth replacement. It would simply help you to understand what you are up against in presenting dental implant treatment plans to such a group and would force you to take a different approach than you would for the group who overwhelmingly expresses displeasure with their RPDs.

SurveyMonkey.com: Use it!

To set up your surveys, the best place to go is www.SurveyMonkey. com. This website makes setting up surveys as easy as apple pie. Another thing that's great about generating surveys through

SurveyMonkey is that it's all electronic, which means you can use your iPad or tablet to have a patient complete a survey while waiting to be seated or while sitting in the operatory waiting to be treated. You guessed it—there is an iPad app for SurveyMonkey, too. You can also poll your fans on social media sites such as your Facebook page, all powered through SurveyMonkey. And because it's all electronic, SurveyMonkey's algorithms have been designed to collect and tabulate your data, and it will keep a running score of what the results are to your questions. For example, 73% of your RPD patients between the ages of 45 and 54 find it difficult to chew with their RPDs in place.

Tailor your marketing efforts to match your research findings

Based on the results from the earlier survey conducted by this *hypothetical dental office*, let's assume we learned the following facts with respect to how your patients feel about their RPDs, how they use them, how long they believe the RPDs should last, and so on:

1 73% in this survey are ages 45–64 and have had their prostheses for 5–7 years.
2 69% in this survey said they tolerate their RPDs.
3 51% in this survey said their RPDs move when they chew, and 48% also said food gets trapped beneath their RPDs.
4 70% in this survey said their RPD improves their smile.
5 48% in this survey believe their RPDs should last between 16 and 20 years.
6 68% in this survey said they wear RPDs to bed at night.
7 39% in this survey said they use denture adhesive to stabilize their RPDs.

Now that we have tabulated the data and have researched the RPD patients to gain a sense of their circumstance and how they feel about their prostheses, the time is now to begin reaching out to these patients. One office might draft a short letter, while another may choose instead to construct a postcard. Either will do for this project.

Box 6.3 Example letter to RPD patients designed to begin dialog.

Dear Patient [personalize],

Please accept this as a routine courtesy follow-up. Our intent is to be sure your removable partial denture continues to function to your satisfaction. If your partial denture fits well and allows you to chew your food properly, please disregard this letter.

If your partial denture is malfunctioning by moving when you chew or allowing food get beneath it, I encourage you to schedule an appointment for a complementary evaluation. An old or loose partial denture that causes you to avoid certain healthy foods is a sacrifice not worth making.

We hope you are completely satisfied with your oral health. If for any reason you have concerns, please contact our office for a complementary evaluation. I'm confident we can either repair or replace your partial denture with a solution that will allow you to function well.

Sincerely,
Dr. Implant Dentist

The key is to use the data from your research to influence the wording of your correspondence.

Nearly 70% said they "tolerate" their RPD, about half this group believes their RPD should last as much as "20 years," and over half this group said they know their RPD "moves" when they chew their food. These are the RPD known hot buttons.

The letter example in Box 6.3 broaches the subject of the partial denture and encourages the patient to speak up if they are, in any way, experiencing issues with their RPD. Note also that the letter encourages the patient to come in for a complimentary examination and consultation. This letter should go out to this group of patients at least two to four times each year. It is only a matter of time before such patients within this group realize there may be a solution to their problems.

Automate your marketing correspondence

This is a good time to make another important point. Sending out marketing letters and postcards to your targeted patient base can be administered and carried out manually by you and your staff on a monthly basis, but I don't recommend it. Pay a professional to stuff, seal and stamp your envelopes, and utilize your time and your staff members' time to do what you do best. I have found that, at best, offices are able to carry out these steps manually for about 3 months before the day-to-day office chaos takes priority or staff turnover leaves this duty unfilled and the effort comes to a halt.

Automation is your friend. Design the process, write the letters for each of the missing-teeth categories, have your lawyer draft a "business associate agreement" to be signed by your print shop for HIPAA reasons, and then give your list of patient names and addresses only, and your credit card to the print shop to send out this correspondence on a regular basis. You need a print shop that is capable of personalizing each letter and mailing your letters out on predetermined dates throughout the year. This way, you don't have to think about it and the job still gets done.

Define your missing teeth demographics

In order to hit your target, you must first understand what is possible. Do you know how many adult missing teeth your patient base represents? Is it 10,000 missing teeth? Who knows? It could very well be 15,000 or 20,000 missing teeth. You need to find out what this number is. I guarantee you that whatever it is, it will be an eye opener.

You will find that once you know this number, instantaneously, your confidence will reach levels you never knew were possible. Suddenly, you will realize that there are so many of your patients in need of your implant services that even if you began one implant case and complete another, every single day your clinical capacity would still be insufficient to care for the potential dental implant cases in your practice. So, let's begin the process of coming up with this number.

Every one of your patients who are missing teeth should fit into a specific category. Every patient within each of these categories should have a missing teeth total number. Lastly, every category should be represented by a total number of missing teeth, as is, in the *Edentulism 1 arch* section of Table 6.1. The 6 patients listed on this abbreviated list represent a total of 112 missing teeth.

Not only have we gathered a total number of missing teeth in this practice, but we have also defined how many missing teeth there are in each category. There are a total of 371 missing teeth among this

Table 6.1 There are five of six missing-teeth categories listed on this abbreviated patient record.

Missing-teeth chart					
Edentulism 1 arch	**Edentulism 2 arches**	**FPD**	**RPD**	**Anterior missing**	**Total all categories**
Lisa Jones—18	Andrea Scott—32	Sherry Lee—4	Jose Lopez—3	Sam Vito—2	
Gary Jackson—16	Mary Lee—32	Lisa Smith—1	Doug Lewis—1	Will Hines—14	
Marie Nguyen—22	Sheryl Tucker—32	Steve Kelly—4	Helen Davis—3	Allen Hadeed—5	
Andrea Lee—19	Seth Levine—32	Lisa Wilson—6	Harlene Toe—8	Jon Phillips—1	
John Smith—20	Chris Frank—32	Tom Jacobs—3	Joe Emery—2	Tonya Harris—4	
Jose Jackson—17	Lee Williams—32	Fay Nguyen—3	April Lee—1	Sandra Drew—2	
Total—112	Total—192	Total—21	Total—18	Total—28	Total 371 (30 pts)

limited number of 30 patients, and for instance, there are 18 missing teeth among the group of 6 RPD patients. Now we're on to something.

Obviously, we can't outline the total list of missing-teeth patients here, but with just a partial list of 30 patients from this practice, we have a very telling target. This is the type of data that positioned Mr. David Cook to know what a new Blockbuster's potential would be or, furthermore, if that prospective new location should never be opened in the first place. The numbers don't lie.

To reach your greatest potential in implant dentistry, you need to understand the numbers. You might presently perform 100 implants each year with a goal to perform 300, for example. Yet when you define your numbers in-depth, you might discover your true potential is really 500 implants annually. Once you understand the numbers, you then chip away at that number week by week, month by month, and year by year through smart internal and external marketing efforts. As the saying goes, "Anyone can eat an elephant one bite at a time."

The numbers don't lie

Follow the guidelines in this chapter for segmenting your database, coupled with the tactical approaches defined in Chapter 1 Visual aids and verbal skills, and it is reasonable to expect a specific segment of your patient base, such as the RPD wearers, to accept your dental implant treatment recommendations at very high closing ratios. In a 2011 article, Dr. Roger P. Levin suggested that with the proper tools in place, including a proficient *implant treatment coordinator*, your dental implant case acceptance can be as high as 90% (Levin, 2011b). I agree completely.

Over the course of a 12- to 18-month period, it is reasonable for a practice with 223 RPD patients of record, such as with the Box 6.1 RPD Patient Database Query, to treat at least 15% of the 223 patients (or 33 patients) with dental implants. Since each RPD patient represents an average of 5.6 missing teeth in this practice, approximately 185 dental implants will be required to replace the missing teeth for these patients.

Please understand that the 15% does not represent the case acceptance rate. The case acceptance rate should be closer to 80–90%. Therefore, to gain acceptance from these RPD patients, the dentist would need to present to 37–41 RPD patients and have 33 patients (or 90%) accept treatment. Treating 33 RPD patients with dental implants within a period of 12–18 months is very realistic.

Now, let's assume these patients accepting the implant treatment plans will conservatively pay a fee of $1,850 for the implant surgery and $1,800 for the restoration or a total of $3,650 per implant. Obviously, this doesn't take into account additional fees required for such procedures as bone and soft tissue grafting. For other patients, a $25,000+ full arch TeethXpress procedure may be necessary. On average, each patient will spend reasonably more to replace their missing teeth with dental implants.

From this very small segment of the practice, we're now looking at approximately $675,250 in implant surgical placements and implant restorations alone. If you only surgically place implants or only restore implants, the numbers are still extremely favorable.

If you are a surgical specialist, how often do you receive 185 dental implant referrals from one dentist over the course of 12–18 months?

Probably not very often. And this number represents only a small segment of the dentist's practice.

If you are a restorative dentist only (no surgery), how often do you generate 185 implant sites for restoration from within a very small segment of your practice over the course of a 12–18-month period? Unless you have internal marketing systems in place, I'm guessing there is room to increase your implant restorative number significantly.

Build rapport year-round

In my lifetime, I've had both bad and good credit, and as long as my credit is good, the credit card companies are very nice to me. They raise my credit limits and reduce my interest rates. My banks tells me how special I am, makes offers of preapproved personal and business loans, and encourages me to use their cash for home improvements. The manufacturer of my 5-year-old automobile sends me birthday greetings and a catalog of their latest model year, with a "0.00%" interest rate offer on the purchase of a new vehicle.

Why do they go through this effort? It is because these companies understand the value in an established relationship and that it is far more cost-effective to target current customers than to establish a new customer relationship. My automobile manufacture understands, at some point, chances are very good that I will have a need for a new car.

As long as your goal is to replace their missing teeth with dental implants—and it should be—you need to begin treating these individuals like close friends. Yes, you should send them marketing letters that speaks to their clinical needs but send them birthday cards, Mother's and Father's Day cards, Happy Anniversary recognitions, Thanksgiving greetings, and so on as well. I call these "white-glove" acknowledgements.

Assign this effort to your implant coordinator. It is her/his job to see to it that you sign the cards. Each one of these patients is contacted four to six times per year with a friendly greeting or gesture from your office. When these patients do eventually visit your office and complain about their partial denture being too loose or that an abutment tooth has broken and you give them all the valid reasons that it is now time to replace their missing teeth with an implant-supported prosthesis, followed by your presentation of a $5,000 or a $50,000 treatment plan, there may be other barriers, but trust won't be one of them. You will also notice an increase in your new patient referrals among this group. White-glove acknowledgments are powerful.

Target each demographic in your database for implants

Establishing missing-teeth categories is important. You need to understand where your targets are before you can hit them. Once you have established each category (as demonstrated in Box 6.4), add each of your patients with missing teeth to the category that best represents their most dominant need. If the patient wears a maxillary RPD and a mandibular complete denture, that patient should most likely be grouped with your *edentulous mandible* marketing list.

When you target a specific segment of your patient database, you can speak to this demographic in a way that represents their explicit concerns. You are suddenly speaking their language. And anytime you speak the language of your targeted audience, you instantly gain rapport.

The self-conscious, emotional-buying decisions affecting the 60-year-old denture-wearing patient is much different from the 25-year-old patient who has congenitally missing maxillary lateral incisors,

Box 6.4 Each of these eight categories should have its own letter.

Missing-teeth categories to target

1 Removable partial denture (RPD)
2 Fixed partial denture (FPD)
3 Anterior missing teeth
4 Posterior missing teeth
5 Edentulous mandible—denture
6 Edentulous maxilla—denture
7 Fully edentulous—dentures
8 Missing teeth—no prosthesis

which is different from the 43-year-old removable partial-denture-wearing patient. Managing your database by compartmentalizing your missing teeth patients allows you to routinely speak to the specific concerns and emotions of each group. Do this and a consistent flow of case acceptance will come without delay.

There are more than 44 million adults suffering from at least one quadrant of posterior missing teeth (Misch, 2007). In 1965, the average person could expect to live to 65. Today, the average individual can expect to reach the age of 80, and a very good percentage will live several years longer. My father celebrated his 92nd birthday in 2015 and drives his own car to visit his 95-year-old brother.

These patients are in your practice. You have to locate such patients and offer them your dental implant services because dental implants are not only good for their oral health; they are good for their overall health. Should a 65-year-old healthy woman be presented a $25,000 treatment plan to replace her missing teeth with dental implants? If such a treatment plan is in the best interest of the patient's health, I say absolutely! No one should be forced to spend the remaining 20 or so years of their life wearing a denture and maintaining a diet that limits what they can eat with an unstable denture. Let this be their choice, but always give them the option. It is the patient's right to understand the options.

Reactivate your inactive patients

This type of target marketing will also help you realize how many patients of record are inactive. As you audit your records, you will find that many of your patients have relocated, sadly enough others have passed away, and unfortunately some have found another dentist.

But your greatest potential for growth rests in those inactive patients who have simply fallen by the wayside for no other reason than the fact that they never rescheduled their perio-maintenance or 6-month recare appointments and have been thinking in the back of their minds that they need to call and schedule an appointment but have just neglected to do so. It could be that, 2 years ago, they went through an ugly divorce, were unemployed, fulfilled an 18-month job assignment overseas, or received a denture from you that they now hate and believe there is no solution after the third reline.

There are several reasons why patients become inactive, many of which are superficial. And a large percentage of these patients need dental implants—point being that you will attract implant treatment from inactive patients too. The added benefit of these efforts is that in many instances your inactive patients become active again, making them even more valuable than new patients for one simple reason— these patients already know you. In fact, there are enough inactive patients in your database who trust you, like you, believe you, and still prefer to be treated by you but have simply fallen off the band- wagon for different reasons.

Whatever the set of circumstances were that caused many of your patients to become inactive, those circumstances do not necessarily still negatively impact a certain percentage of these patients today. Time will always bring about a change in one's circumstance. This is why you must routinely and consistently target your patient database for dental implants, especially your inactive patients, before someone else does.

It is impossible to always know which of your patients' circum- stances have changed for the better. But you can be 100% confident in knowing that a reasonable percentage of your patients' circum- stances are always changing in ways that make them far better pros- pects for dental implants (and other oral care) today than they were when you last treated them 3 months ago or 3 years ago.

Drop your buckets where you are

In his 1895 Atlanta Compromise speech, the civil rights leader Booker T. Washington famously told the story of a lost ship having finally been sighted by a friendly vessel after being misplaced at sea for several days. He proceeded to chronicle how the lost ship sent out a message to the friendly vessel, "Water, water, we're dying of thirst!" The friendly ship replied, "Cast down your bucket where you are." The lost ship shouted again, "Water, water, we're dying of thirst!" The friendly ship repeated this advice once again and then a third time. Only after the fourth time of advising the distressed vessel to drop down their buckets into the surrounding water did the captain of the distressed ship do so.

When the captain lifted his buckets, he discovered that they were not full of salt water as he had presumed. It turned out his buckets were full of fresh, sparkling water from the mouth of the Amazon River. The sailor of this lost vessel almost died of thirst not realizing that he and his crew was surrounded by as much digestible water as they needed.

Your practice is no different. You are sitting on as many dental implant cases as you are capable of handling. Recognizing the implant cases that surround you requires that you change your paradigm and pay closer attention to your patients of record. As mentioned before, there are 1249 edentulous sites within the scenario I have laid out for you, most of which are ideal sites for dental implants. In many ways, chances are your practice is no different. All you need is a very small percentage of your patients (from this and other segments that you will define) to accept your well-presented, dental implant treatment plan.

Summary

Database marketing is one of the most predicable ways any dental professional can grow their dental implant business. When specific missing-teeth segments within a practice are systematically targeted for the purposes of treating such patients with dental implants, the results can be quite impressive. No dental implant prospect will trust you more than your pleased patients who have an established track record of accepting dental treatment from you in the past.

For this reason alone, you must understand your missing-teeth demographics all the way down to the number of missing teeth in your practice. This number will not only help you understand your potential, but it will give you a sense of responsibility to help so many more patients to replace their missing teeth in the most effective way possible—with dental implants.

In most practices, dental professionals are surrounded by hundreds and thousands of patients in need of dental implants. Doctors that perform above-average dental implant procedures almost always understand how to target their patient databases.

CHAPTER 7

Internet presence

This may be the last chapter in the book, but please don't mistake it for being insignificant in any way. I have done my best to cut to the chase here because I know there is a very good chance you have little interest in becoming an expert at promoting your dental implant services over the Internet.

You don't have to be an expert to understand that whether your prospective implant patients were referred by a friend or family member or perhaps your office is represented on their dental insurance preferred provider list or whatever other means an implant candidate has used to find you, people will frequently check you out online before they move forward with your services. If you question the veracity of this fact, just think about how often you explore the Internet to aid you in your decision-making process when it comes to learning more about a medical condition, choosing a restaurant, or buying a new vehicle and everything in between.

There was a time in the early 2000s when establishing a meaningful Internet presence was completely optional, and when it came to small business, it was the early adaptors choosing to establish nice websites. Eventually, social media was introduced and Facebook established what is now called a *Like* page for businesses primarily, suddenly giving you the ability to post subjects specific to your dental practice in an online, social environment. And then along

Marketing Implant Dentistry: Attract and Influence Patients to Accept Your Dental Implant Treatment Plan, First Edition. Marcus Hines.
© 2016 John Wiley & Sons, Inc. Published 2016 by John Wiley & Sons, Inc.

came rating sites like Yelp and Angie's List where people could post exactly how they felt about your services, good or bad, for everyone else to see.

Today, in 2015, you *must* have an Internet presence that not only attracts attention, but equally important, garners respect. This includes having a first-rate website that is well optimized, an active social media presence, and, last but not least, very positive online reviews about you and the dental implant services you provide.

Website

Just because you can purchase a generic "Websites-R-Us" template, figure out how to upload images, and describe a dental procedure in two paragraphs or less doesn't mean you are qualified to design your business's website. Oftentimes, it takes multiple conversations to convince some of my clients that a dental website should not be treated like a commodity. In many instances, this will be the first impression the general public will have of your office. Do you want your Internet visitors to pass on your office because your website looks cheap and insufficient?

I don't even encourage you to spend good money on a professional website if it means it will be designed from scratch unless you are one of a very small few who is capable of uploading the required content to make your website complete. Content is king, and in many ways, your content is as important as the aura of your website. No matter how good of a writer you believe you are, it is nearly impossible to write the content for your website in a way that is comprehensive, informative, grammatically correct, and easy to read for the layman viewer.

We have become a society that uses our mobile phones and tablets to not only communicate but to surf the Internet for much of our personal needs. Today more than ever, having a website that is conducive to a mobile device is increasingly important. Today, a practice's website should be capable of being navigated on a mobile device with ease.

Don't fool around with it—just outsource it. Establish a respectable budget and hire a proven dental–medical website developer to do it for you. Who cares that they can have you up and running in a matter of days and still charge you $6,000 or more? In some regards, all professionals get paid this way. Depending on your experience, you can probably numb the patient, lay the flap, and bang out two adjacent posterior implants in a matter of 15–20 minutes. Does that mean your patient should feel cheated by your $4,400 charge for the 30 minutes they sat in your chair? Of course not. The value they receive as a result of your countless hours of training is potentially lifelong. You pay for the web developer's years of experience and expertise, specific to dentistry.

Implant content

The better dental and medical website developers will provide you with comprehensive content on dental implants. Most every topic, including information about bone loss, bone grafting, implant placement, and so on, will be covered to some degree. But no matter how comprehensive the content, you will always need to make your dental implant content your own. In other words, you will do well to elaborate on some of the topics and also add before-and-after images and video testimonials from your satisfied implant patients. No web developer can do this for you.

If you routinely perform full-arch, dental implant-supported prostheses and have documented your cases, make sure you upload these images. If you have before-and-after, esthetic-zone cases that are very appealing to the eye, you will do well to add these images to your website, too. Just leave the surgical content out.

On many occasions, I've seen doctors post gory, surgical videos and images on what should be a patient-friendly website. If this is you, I would encourage you to take them all down. To the patient, there is nothing impressive about your ability to take a blade to someone's gums, expose the bloody jawbone, enter the mouth with a drill, drill a hole, and ratchet in a titanium metal rod. When's the last time you videotaped a third-molar extraction, an endodontic procedure, followed by a crown prep, then posted that video to your patient-friendly website?

You and I know implant surgery is not a painful procedure, but try convincing a patient of that after seeing your video. To the patient, the only thing that's impressive about implant dentistry is the end result. Patients want to know what their teeth replacement will look like and how it will function when you're done.

You are much better off to limit your patient visuals to smile-line, before-and-after images.

Search engine optimization

There are at least three primary search engines that your patients and everyone else not living under a rock use on a daily basis: Google, Bing, and Yahoo. Certainly, you are familiar with these three search engines and probably routinely use at least one of them. When prospective dental implant patients go online and use keywords and keyword phrases such as "implants" or "dental implants" or "implant teeth," and so on, your goal is to have your website come up on the first page in your area. This is called "search engine optimization" (SEO).

The best dental–medical-specific website developers will offer the service of optimizing your website for an additional fee. Take advantage of it. Not to do so would be sort of like buying an S-Class Mercedes-Benz and insisting on changing the oil and performing the manufacturer's recommended maintenance yourself, all in the name of saving a few dollars. Again, these are the professionals and they can put you in the best position for success. They understand what the keyword phrases are for implant dentistry and can work on the back end of your website to optimize such words and phrases for you.

That said, there are steps you can take to aid the process of SEO. The search engines like it when there is fresh activity on your website. This tells the search engine algorithms that your website is active and is not merely taking up space in the cyber world.

Blog

One of the best ways to keep your website fresh and active is to create a *blog*. A blog is great because it allows you to write fresh content on whatever subject you choose. My recommendation is that your office posts a blog about implant dentistry at least once or twice a month. The more you blog the better. This blog can be on whatever dental-related subject that happens to inspire you to write. Certainly, each week, there is a different procedure you perform that interests you enough to post a one- or two-paragraph blog about. My recommendation is that you make the topic of dental implants a part of your weekly blog at least once each month for starters. This will help with your SEO for dental implants.

YouTube

Another very useful tool that will help you in a number of ways, including SEO, is video, and *YouTube*® is the vehicle you will want to use to host your video. Here's the long and the short of it: Google owns YouTube, and therefore, Google's algorithms are set up to favor websites that link YouTube videos back to their business's website. For this reason, it behooves you to create multiple, short, dental implant-related videos; upload these short videos to YouTube; and link your YouTube videos to your website.

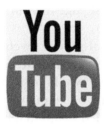

This really is as easy as it sounds. And as easy as it is, you may still choose not to go through this process. If this is the case, ask a young staff member to do it for you. If you have a teenager or 20-something staff member, most likely they will already know what steps to take to make this happen for you. If not, hire your teenage child to do it for you. The part you need to get involved with is having your satisfied dental implant patients agree to go on record (video) with their testimonials.

YouTube is a very, very powerful tool for you. Behind Google, YouTube is the second-largest search engine. What's also fascinating about YouTube is that just like the major social media websites, YouTube is also a community. With YouTube, you have the ability to establish your own "channel" and can encourage viewers to subscribe to this "channel" and receive updated information as you post new implant patient testimonials to it.

For the purposes of growing your dental implant business, be encouraged by the fact that 68% of YouTube viewers want to be entertained and 28% are looking for information, according to James Wedmore, a foremost YouTube authority (Wedmore, 2014). Wedmore says, "Video is excellent for branding and establishing professionalism. Video has the ability to establish you as the authority and give you celebrity status." To this point, I would encourage you to upload two types of videos to YouTube and appropriately position them on your website.

Video type #1: Testimonial videos

The first kind of videos I encourage you to create are patient testimonial videos. The patient testimonial videos should consist of satisfied patients who are willing to go on record with why they believe you are the "world's greatest dental implant doctor," in about 2–3 minutes, tops. Anything longer than 3 minutes should be edited down by extrapolating the most valuable points made during the video. You may find the 5- to 10-minute video quite flattering because it's all about how great you are, but for everyone else, anything longer than 3 minutes and you run the risk of losing the viewer's interest.

To make the testimonial videos, you'll simply need a smart phone and a third-grader's level of understanding on how to upload these testimonial videos to YouTube. The second type of video will require a little more effort on your part and will take more time to produce but will be well worth it.

Video type #2: Treatment/education videos

The second kind of videos I encourage you to create are treatment/ education videos. These are short videos of you speaking in front of the camera about a particular dental implant procedure. For instance, alongside your text description of a full-arch, immediate-occlusal-function procedure, you will also have a video that briefly describes the same procedure. This gives the prospective patient the opportunity to both read the description of the procedure and also to see and hear you describe the procedure.

When done correctly, this will enhance your website's ability to have more influence on visitors. At the end of each video, you should encourage the viewer to go to the section on your website where they can sign up for your *patient implant education seminar*. Now, you are really cooking!

While your testimonial videos can go as long as 2–3 minutes, the treatment/education video should be kept to less than 1 minute.

Google Adwords

Google Adwords is a great way to advertise on the web. The prospective dental implant patient does a Google search for "implant dentist" in your area and up pops your name/office as one of the top listings on the search engine. Granted, it that this is not an organic listing, since you paid for it, it's actually an advertisement. That said, it's clever because it doesn't look like an "ad"; it looks like a listing.

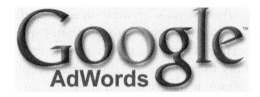

What's nice about Google Adwords is that you are charged only when someone clicks on your website listing. When you set up your Google Adwords account, you establish a daily budget, and once that budget is met, your ad is no longer listed for that day. You can set the budget for as much or as little as you like.

Let's say you would like to budget $600 per month to advertise your dental implant business through Google Adwords. Assuming you figure 30 days in a month on average, your daily budget will be $20. If Google will charge, say, $0.70 per click for certain keyword searches in your area, such a budget represents up to 28 leads that can be pushed to your website or landing page or where ever you choose to have your traffic flow to. Again, you only pay for the amount of people that click your ad. This is great because if only four people click your ad on any given day, based on the above assumed per-click fee, you only pay $2.80.

Google Adwords has the ability to bring you traffic, but your advertising will only be as effective as the destination that you send prospective dental implant patients to. If your website is of poor quality and the content is incomplete, your traffic will not manifest into dental implant patients, and the visitors will continue on with their Google searches until they find what they are looking for in a dental implant practice. If you have great video testimonials of satisfied implant patients, a dental implant-specific landing page that entices the prospective implant patient to take the next step, or a great dental implant educational content that intrigues its readers, your Google Adwords ad can be extremely productive.

Landing page (or squeeze page)

Every dental or specialty practice should have a comprehensive office website. A *landing page* (also known as a squeeze page) should not be mistaken for a practice's website. Describing your practice and outlining each of the procedures you offer is not the intent of a landing page.

A landing page is somewhat like a miniwebsite with its own URL that focuses on a small niche service (or product). Your landing page will only include information about one procedure in particular—implant dentistry. With a landing page, you can choose to be even more specific within the grand scheme of implant dentistry and therefore can choose to limit your content to full-arch, dental implant-supported prostheses.

A landing page can be a very effective tool for your practice because it hones in on a specific topic that the prospective patient is interested in. And because the landing page is so focused, you can really optimize the page for a particular service that you are promoting. This will allow you to strategically use certain keywords, all of which are good for SEO. And the better your SEO is for a particular procedure—implant dentistry, TeethXpress®, implant dentures, etc.—the greater the chances are that your landing page will come up on the first one or two pages of a search engine. Of course, you can always send your Google AdWords traffic to your landing page as well.

I won't get into how to create a landing page here; there are too many white papers, manuals, and online resources that can offer you the information, in addition to simply hiring a credible web developer to create it for you. But I will tell you that a landing page is one of the best ways to promote your dental implant procedures online.

You can create a landing page to promote your implant patient education seminars, for example. Such a site should be designed to draw the reader in and allow the reader to register for your free patient education seminars right there on your landing page. A different landing page might discuss the benefits and process of replacing a lower denture with an implant-supported fixed prosthesis. It should be easy for the patient to register for a free consultation appointment directly from your landing page.

Another landing page can address dental implants for the esthetic zone only, display before-and-after images, and show successfully treated patient testimonials, followed by a download of a free booklet titled "Ten Questions Every Patient Should Ask Their Dental-Implant Provider Before Accepting the Treatment Plan," for example. And such a guide might address some of the most common issues patients should be aware of when receiving dental implants in the esthetic zone. The fact that you have gone to this extent and are providing the information for free speaks volumes to the prospective patient and indirectly promotes your practice for this type of procedure.

I think you get the point. Landing pages should be highly niche but should have a call to action and lead prospective patients into taking the next step, which is registering for an appointment or downloading additional information, which brings them even closer to being treated with dental implants in your office.

Social media

It still makes me laugh whenever I hear the story of Willie Sutton, who in the early to mid-1900s was a serial bank robber. He was estimated to have stolen more than $2 million over the course of his 40-year criminal career. As urban legend would have it, when Willie Sutton was asked, "Why do you rob banks?" His reply was, "Because that's where the money is." To this day, every time I hear that story it makes me chuckle, even when I tell it. If this whole dental implant thing doesn't work out for you, I'm not encouraging you to try your hand at robbing banks. Willie Sutton might have been good at it, but he also spent half of his adult life in jail.

But as a healthcare provider and business owner, you should get involved with social media. Why? Because that's where your professional colleagues and prospective dental implant patients are. For this reason alone, you, too, should be there.

LinkedIn
Of all the social media sites available, pound for pound from a business prospective, LinkedIn is my favorite—hands down. From a business-to-business (B-to-B) standpoint, I am most active on LinkedIn and will unabashedly take this opportunity to say that if you like what you

have read so far in my book Marketing Implant Dentistry and you are interested in maintaining a professional relationship with me, I would like to connect with you on LinkedIn. I can be found on LinkedIn at https://www.linkedin.com/in/marcushines. When you send the request to connect, if you would add a brief note on your thoughts of my book, I would be most appreciative.

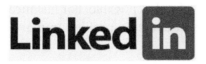

Now, let's get back to business. While most of the popular social media sites were designed for the average person to "socialize," LinkedIn is unique in the sense that it is all about business networking. There are more than 300 million registered LinkedIn users (Wagner, 2014). This makes LinkedIn the world's largest professional social media network by far.

Speakers and clinicians on LinkedIn

If you lecture to other dental professionals, have written a dental book and want to sell more copies, have authored dental articles and case reports, consult dental professionals, teach implant dentistry to dental professionals, or offer any of these or other expert professional services, it behoves you to solidify your presence on LinkedIn. But you don't need to be a world-class clinician or presenter in order to have a complete LinkedIn profile. If you are a surgical specialist who counts on referrals from multiple dentists, a prosthodontist specializing in implant restorations, or a general practitioner who places and/or restores dental implants, you, too, would be wise to have an impressive LinkedIn profile and to use LinkedIn as a form to connect and dialogue with other clinicians that you would benefit from working with.

You will find that setting up your LinkedIn account is self-explanatory, such as your contact information and your educational background. With that said, there are certain sections that many professionals take way too lightly or skip over altogether. Be as comprehensive about your professional background and clinical experience as possible.

LinkedIn summary outline

One section you should not ignore is the "Summary." This section is called a *Summary* for a reason, so avoid telling your life story here. However, if you are particularly well trained, experienced, or passionate about performing certain dental procedures (hint: implant dentistry), be sure to include it here in one to two paragraphs. In some cases, two paragraphs may not do you justice given your CV. Just keep in mind that you should be as brief as possible. For instance Figure 7.1 demonstrates my professional LinkedIn profile summary.

LinkedIn experience outline

The next section in LinkedIn is for professional experiences and is another section that should not be taken lightly. Job and business/practice ownership experiences go here. This is pretty cool because

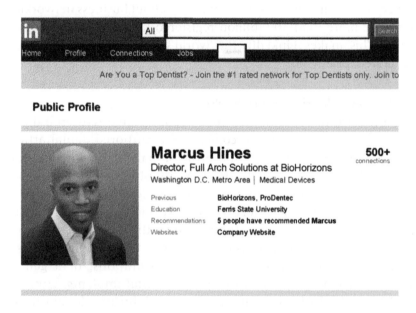

Figure 7.1 Your LinkedIn Summary should be clear, concise and effective at demonstrating your expertise to the viewer of your profile.

LinkedIn's algorithms are such that when certain keyword searches are performed by your colleagues, you stand a good chance of being discovered when your *Experience* sections are completed properly. If you are a surgical specialist, you'll want to include plenty of keywords about the types of dental implant procedures you perform, including anterior immediate implant provisionals. If you conduct dental implant courses, or say, hands-on training in advanced bone grafting, you will do well to include these terms within your Experience section also. The goal is to be discovered on LinkedIn and online.

LinkedIn publications listings

There is even a publications section on LinkedIn. If you have written a book, published articles, or performed certain documented research, this is the place for it. Don't be humble. Listing as many publications as you have generated will only add to your credibility with other professionals and prospective patients.

Surgical specialists on LinkedIn

Professional networking doesn't get any better than LinkedIn when it comes to social media. This is why the surgical specialist must have an impressive profile on LinkedIn. When general dentists are seeking out certain experiences and characteristics in a surgeon for the purposes of referring implant patients, you want your profile to appear. Once your profile comes up in their search, you are highly favored to win the attention of that dentist and ultimately his or her patient referral. It also behooves you to join dental implant-related groups and routinely dialogue with other members. As long as you speak intelligently on any given topic and avoid petty back-and-forth opinionated debates, your viewpoints won't go unnoticed and ultimately will lead to professional relationship opportunities.

Being discovered by patients on LinkedIn

While LinkedIn is much more of a B-to-B social network versus a business-to-consumer (B-to-C)-driven social network, like Facebook, prospective implant patients will Google your name after being referred by a friend, hearing your radio advertisement, or receiving a promotional correspondence in the mail. If your LinkedIn page is well optimized, your LinkedIn profile stands a greater chance of coming up high on their Google search, ideally on the first page. Having each of your dental implant credentials and experiences listed in good fashion will be quite impressive to any prospective patient who discovers you on LinkedIn.

When you present a prospective implant patient with, say, a $25,000 treatment plan, it is reasonable to expect that patient to do their own due diligence of you and your experience. When the patient performs a Google search of your name, your LinkedIn profile will most likely appear on the first page. In this situation LinkedIn will benefit you the most when your impressive experience is fully represented.

Facebook

As of October 2014, there were more than 1.35 billion monthly active Facebook users (Smith, 2014). I can't think of any good reason a small business owner, such as a dental practice, should not be on Facebook. When it comes to your business, you must always look for opportunities to network, and if nothing else, your patients are on Facebook, which means you, too, should be on Facebook.

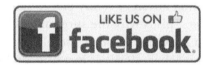

The main component of Facebook that might benefit your business is the Facebook business *Like* page. I like to think of the *Like* page as being a miniblog site that resides within Facebook. Here, you have the opportunity to post images and share short messages about oral health and current events. You can post an excerpt from your website about dental implants and include a link back to your website for those interested enough to read the detailed write-up on the subject. You might also post a fun image of you and your friends at an NFL tailgate party, for instance. This is a powerful tool because everyone on Facebook who has chosen to *Like* your page in the past will receive each of your Facebook posts, giving them the opportunity to read your write-ups or view your videos and so on.

If for some reason you still can't tell—and as I've stated before in this book—let me be explicit: *I am a very big proponent of implant patient education seminars.* And Facebook is a great tool for you because it allows you to consistently send out invitations for your patient education seminars each and every month to everyone who has *Liked* your *Like* page and to your Facebook "friends." You can even establish private groups on Facebook that allow you to invite *only* dental and medical professionals to your group. You can then use these groups to network and engage in clinical discussions with respect to implant dentistry and other procedures.

Yes, you will advertise your implant patient education seminars on the radio; yes, you will send out postcards to promote your patient education seminars to your targeted patient base; yes, you will promote your patient education seminars to medical professionals—all aside from Facebook—but if you're wise, you will also target your list of 500+ Facebook "followers." Before you know it, of the 20 people who attended your most recent implant patient education seminar, five of them attended as a result of receiving a Facebook promotion from your office. No such results are possible without attaining a following on your Facebook *Like* page.

Your goal should be to get to 500 or more Facebook *Likes* as rapidly as possible. How do you do this? Taking an organic approach is ideal. Once your Facebook *Like* page has been established and if you're already on Facebook, immediately send out a request to all of your Facebook "friends" and request that they *Like* your Facebook page. Facebook makes it easy for you to do this systematically.

Next, you will need to ask your patients who are on Facebook to go to your website and *Like* your Facebook page. Most people don't mind doing this at the request of a business they are familiar with or are interested in. Even before you start dental procedures, ask your patients if they are on Facebook. When they say yes, tell them you are attempting to build your presence on Facebook and would very much appreciate it if they would take a quick second before you start the procedure to go to your website and *Like* your Facebook page. And since most people use a smart phone, they can easily go to your website while waiting to be treated. Chances are good that your patients are already browsing Facebook while waiting to be treated anyway.

Twitter

Many of your patients are also using Twitter. According to an October 2014 report by Digital Marketing Ramblings, there are 284 million active monthly users of Twitter. While Twitter may not offer you the opportunities to directly promote to your target audience in the same way that a Facebook business *Like* page can and Facebook pay-per-click advertising does, Twitter is a social media tool that virtually no oral healthcare provider should ignore. For the purposes of running a dental practice, think of Twitter as being a community billboard of sorts.

How does Twitter work?

In a nutshell, it will take you less than 5 minutes to establish a Twitter account, and before you know it, you are able to start posting tweets and following me on Twitter at @MarcusHines. A "tweet" is the term used for a message posted on Twitter. On Twitter, you "follow" others who are also on Twitter, and you hope others will choose to follow you. Using only 140 characters or less, you can express your thoughts, post images, or share your experiences with everyone who chooses to follow you.

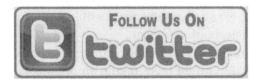

One way to guarantee that no one will follow you for long is to make most every tweet about a dental-related topic such as implants. Here's the reality; unless you are a dental society seeking dentists as your Twitter followers, your average follower is just not interested in reading so many posts about dentistry. Instead, routine posts about things the general public will find interesting, funny, or relatable are in order here. The key is to "be human." There will be plenty opportunities to tweet about dental-related topics.

Perhaps, you were enjoying the Oscars. Why not post a quick tweet about it? You might post something like "Ellen DeGeneres is hilarious at the Oscars LOL!," or if you are a Detroit Lions' fan, like me, you might say, "Lions just may be Super Bowl bound if Stafford avoids throwing picks and Suh plays with reckless abandonment!!!" I know the Lions and Super Bowl aren't usually found in the same sentence, but what can I say, I like to dream big!

I agree with how authors Dr. Jason Lipscomb and Mr. Stephen Knight put it in their book, *Social Media for Dentists 3.0*, "Whatever you do, do not begin tweeting about being a dentist and talking about your practice. You will quickly become an outcast—you need to be tactful" (Lipscomb & Knight, 2012).

Building your followership

Routinely ask your patients to follow you on Twitter. Post a sign in your office with each of your social media sites listed. You will also want to actively ask patients to follow you on Twitter.

It's also a good idea to follow your adult patients on twitter as well. Following your patients will give you great insight to their interests and experiences since people freely share this information on twitter. Oftentimes, you will have opportunities to comment on your patients' lighthearted posts that you share a common interest in, using this platform. The more you can have your patients see you as a normal person, the greater the likelihood they will recommend you to their inner circle.

What's Twitter got to do with implants?

People share their personal dental experiences on Twitter all the time. Someone might tweet, "I'm convinced my dentist is a miracle worker! She fixed my tooth and it didn't even hurt!" or "Had my wisdom teeth pulled and still a little woozy, but surprisingly no pain!" or "My implant tooth looks amazing! Thanks, Dr. Smith!!!"

Sometimes people are just looking for a new dentist. It could be they are fed up with their current dentist or maybe they have just relocated to your town and need a dentist. The prospective patient may send out a tweet that says "Can anyone recommend a good dentist in Washington, DC?" Since I happen to be very pleased with my dentist, I might respond to this tweet by saying, "@JohnDoe Dr. Daniel Hines is an amazing DC dentist, right off the redline!!! www.TakomaParkDentist.com." If the prospective patient is 35 years or older, the chances are very good that they are missing at least one or more teeth, have failing bridge work, or have teeth that need to be removed and replaced with dental implants. You've just attracted a new implant patient through Twitter.

Once you have established your Twitter page with multiple posts on no particular subject, it is totally acceptable to begin occasionally posting about some of your dental profession-related topics. For instances, you might put up a post that says something like, "So proud of the results we achieved for my 70-year-old dental implant patient whose denture no longer worked! Check out these before/after pics! Love to help people smile/eat!!!"

Unfortunately, not all dental experiences posted to Twitter are positive. For instance, your patient might post, "My dentist charges me a 'no-show fee,' so how bout he pays me when he's 1 hr late, really Dr. Smith???" or "I hate getting my teeth cleaned. So painful!!!"

Having an active Twitter account is the best way to understand what conversations people are having about dentistry. Some of these people are, no doubt, your patients. Therefore, now as much as ever, it behooves you to keep your patients satisfied since the chances are good they will share their experiences with their followers and the Twitter community. And when you recognize a patient who chooses to share their unpleasing experience with the world (involving your practice), use that opportunity to make good on it by contacting the patient and working it out.

Instagram

Instagram is another social media site you can expect to find your patients hanging out on. As of March 2014, there were 200 million active Instagram users, according to *Digital Marketing Ramblings*. Instagram has 90 million monthly users who post 40 million photos each and every day. And as of late 2013, 25% of *Fortune 500* companies were using Instagram.

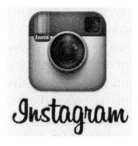

Instagram is great for your business because it's about posting images. Before-and-after images of your implant cases are perfect for Instagram. Pictures taken during your implant patient education seminars may also be posted to your Instagram site. But this is a fun place to hang out, too, so don't forget to post those pictures from your birthday celebrations and Halloween and Christmas parties or of you and your staff member caught on camera having fun. You may even choose to post pictures from your family vacation.

Of all the social media websites, Instagram is by far the easiest to maintain, and because it is owned by Facebook, sharing Instagram posts with your Facebook page is effortless. Every dental implant practice should have an active Instagram page because this social media site not only allows you to showcase your best work, but it lets your patients see the human side of you as well.

Rating sites

From the moment that your patients call you to schedule an appointment through the time they have been successfully treated, more than ever before, how you serve your patients can make all the difference in how you are perceived online. Be careful. These days, people don't mind posting negative reviews online about you and your business for the world to see. Equally important, prospective dental implant patients will go online to check you out in a heartbeat, just to find out what others think about your bedside manner and services before they even agree to schedule an appointment or accept your treatment plan.

Yelp.com, AngiesList.com, HealthGrades.com, ZocDoc.com, DrOogle.com, and other online rating websites are not to be ignored. Angie's List (Figure 7.2) is publicly traded, has a very large advertising budget to attract new members, and promotes the fact they are truly the consumer's advocate.

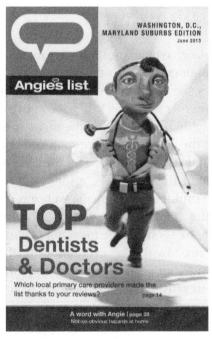

Figure 7.2 Each month Angie's List sends a magazine with helpful hints and local business reviews to its members.

The best thing you can do with such a site is to be proactive. Make sure that if you have a profile posted on any of these sites, your profile is complete and includes meaningful details about your dental implant background. You will also want to be proactive in asking any of your successfully treated implant patients to go to these sites and post a positive review about their experience in your office. Now, when your prospective implant patients are considering spending $25,000–$50,000 at your office and decide to check you out at Yelp.com or AngiesList.com, their confidence in you will only be heightened and the decision to move forward with treatment will be made easier.

I hesitate to give an in-depth analysis here on any one particular review site for reasons that some of these sites have their own fair share of unfavorable reviews and others are quite fluid in their designs. Regardless of this fact, online reviews are here to stay and you must be willing to manage this aspect of your Internet presence. Managing your online reviews well, with respect to your dental implant business, can help lead to positive responses from prospective implant patients.

Summary

In today's marketplace, where prospective patients are using mobile devices and smart phones to search the Internet and do their own due diligence before selecting a healthcare provider, it is important that you have a prominent Internet presence. When it comes to implant dentistry, your goal is to be highly ranked among the three major search engines. In order to achieve this, you must have solid content on your website that is informative and can be optimized for ideal keyword searches.

It is also important that you have a solid and active social media presence. There are multiple social media websites you can use to help benefit your practice. LinkedIn is most significant for B-to-B net-working, and Facebook is one of the most important social media sites for a B-to-C presence. Lastly, be ever mindful of what people are saying about you and your services online. More importantly, be pro-active by asking your satisfied implant patients to go online and post a positive testimonial about their experience in your office on sites like Yelp.com, AngiesList.com, HealthGrades.com, and others.

Conclusion

My hope is that you have found Marketing Implant Dentistry to be well worth the time you have set aside to read it. More importantly, I hope you will take action and help more of your patients recognize the enormous benefits of choosing to replace their missing teeth with dental implants.

We can't ignore the fact that some patients simply do not have the resources to pay for implant dentistry, because it is a reality. But, so many more patients refuse treatment based on a lackluster dental implant treatment plan presentation. Far too frequently, dental professionals fall short of convincing the patient that their money is best spent restoring their oral health with dental implants. As a result, the patient often spends their hard-earned dollars on other things that bring them greater perceived value such as a large screen smart television, a lavish vacation or an upgrade to a two-year old luxury sedan.

Your desire to have more of your patients accept your dental implant treatment plans requires good use of visual aids and verbal skills that will resonate and make a profound impact. Because implant dentistry is, by all intents and purposes, an elective procedure that frequently costs significantly more than traditional methods of tooth replacement, giving each patient a compelling rationale for your recommended dental implant treatment plan is essential.

Through Marketing Implant Dentistry, I have attempted to share multiple examples of proven tools that will help you attract prospective implant patients to your practice, including patient education seminars and forging opportunities to network with your physician colleagues. Even if you do nothing more than look within your accumulated database of patients with missing teeth, followed by thoroughly educating them on the benefits of replacing their missing teeth

Marketing Implant Dentistry: Attract and Influence Patients to Accept Your Dental Implant Treatment Plan, First Edition. Marcus Hines.

with dental implants, you will soon discover the large volume of patients that will move forward with your implant treatment recommendations.

Implant dentistry is such a profound service, capable of solving many problems for so many people that it should not be difficult to deliver a compelling rationale, and have it resonate, as long as you first thoroughly understand your patient, their complaints, concerns and desires.

Steve Jobs said, "We don't get a chance to do that many things... Life is brief, and then you die, you know? And we've all chosen to do this with our lives..." Since time is the most precious commodity we have, the time to act is now. Take action on advancing the way you market implant dentistry and you will position your practice to help more patients make one of the best healthcare decisions of their lives.

Works cited

Associated-Press. (2014). *Colorado Sees Its Best Recreational Marijuana Pot Sales in June*. New York: OregonLive.com.

Bagley, III, D. S., & Reese, E. J. (1988). *Beyond Selling*. Cupertino, CA: Meta Publications, Inc.

Covey, D. S. (1989). *The 7 Habits of Highly Effective People*. New York: Simon & Schuster, Inc.

Douglass, C. W., Shih, A., & Ostry, L. (2002). Will there be a need for complete dentures in the United States in 2020? *Journal of Prosthetic Dentistry*, **87**, 5–8.

Edelman, R. (May 21, 2012). The Truth About Money (D. Liebenson, Interviewer).

Graslie, S. (2013). *Blockbuster Fades Out, But Some Zombie Stores Will Live On*. Washington, DC: NPR.

Levato, D. C. (2014). Choosing the Right Dental Practice Management Software. *Inside Dentistry*, **10**, 22–25.

Levin, R. P. (2011a). *Increase Implant Case Acceptance*. Chicago, IL: AAID.

Levin, R. P. (2011b). *Why an Implant Treatment Coordinator Is Critical to Your Implant Success*. Chicago, IL: AAID.

Lipscomb, J., & Knight, S. (2012). *Social Media for Dentists 3.0*. Richmond, VA: Social Media for Dentists.

McAnally, D. J. (2013). *The Dentist's Unfair Advantage*. Lexington, KY: Dr. James R. McAnally.

Misch, D. C. (2007). *Contemporary Implant Dentistry* (3rd ed.). Maryland Heights, MO: Mosby Elsevier.

Misch, L.S., & Misch, C. E. (1991). Denture satisfaction: a patient's perspective. *International Journal of Oral Implantology*, **7**, 43–48.

Moody, J. (2011). Personalize the Practice with More Digital Tools. *Dental Economics*, **101**, http://www.dentaleconomics.com/articles/print/volume-101/issue-10/technology-needs/personalizing-the-practice-with-more-digital-tools.html (accessed May 11, 2015).

Moon, Y. (2010). *Different: Escaping the Competitive Herd*. New York: Crown Publishing Group.

Marketing Implant Dentistry: Attract and Influence Patients to Accept Your Dental Implant Treatment Plan, First Edition. Marcus Hines.
© 2016 John Wiley & Sons, Inc. Published 2016 by John Wiley & Sons, Inc.

Newport, F. (2010). *Most Americans Take Doctor's Advice Without Second Opinion.* Washington, DC: Gallup Well-Being.

NHTSA. (2014). *Thirty Years of Saving Lives: Happy Birthday to the Airbag.* Washington, DC: NHTSA.

Resnik, R. (July/August 2014). CBCT—Not So Incidental Findings. *Implant Practice*, 28–29.

Roberts, R. (June 2013). A Chat with the Most Trusted Woman on Television (L. Vaccariello, Interviewer).

Smith, C. (2014). *Digital Marketing Ramblings.* Boston, MA: DMR Publisher.

Wagner, K. (2014). *LinkedIn Hits 300 Million Users Amid Mobile Push.* San Francisco, CA: Mashable.

Wedmore, J. (2014). *Video Traffic Academy.* Orange County, CA: Inspired Marketing – Video Traffic Academy.

Wikipedia. (June 9, 2014). Wikipedia Elevator Pitch. Retrieved August 26, 2014, from Wikipedia: http://en.wikipedia.org/wiki/Elevator_pitch (accessed April 22, 2015).

Index

Marketing Implant Dentistry: Attract and Influence Patients to Accept Your Dental Implant Treatment Plan, First Edition. Marcus Hines.
© 2016 John Wiley & Sons, Inc. Published 2016 by John Wiley & Sons, Inc.

Printed and bound by CPI Group (UK) Ltd, Croydon, CR0 4YY

03/04/2024

14479080-0001